# A POCKET GYNAECOLOGY

# A POCKET GYNAECOLOGY

By

## STANLEY G. CLAYTON
M.D., M.S.(Lond.), F.R.C.S., F.R.C.O.G.

*Professor of Obstetrics and Gynaecology,
King's College Hospital Medical School,
University of London*

*Hon-Consulting Obstetric
and Gynaecological Surgeon
Queen Charlotte's Hospital and
Chelsea Hospital for Women*

*Sometime Examiner to the Universities of London, Oxford,
Cambridge, Birmingham, Wales and Dublin, and to
the Royal College of Obstetricians
and Gynaecologists*

SEVENTH EDITION

With 17 Illustrations

## CHURCHILL LIVINGSTONE
Edinburgh and London
1972

First Edition . . . . . 1948

Second Edition . . . . 1952

Third Edition . . . . . 1956

Fourth Edition . . . . 1961

Fifth Edition . . . . . 1965

Sixth Edition . . . . . 1967

   ,,     ,,    Reprinted . 1969

Seventh Edition . . . . 1972

Standard Book Number
0 443 00926 0

Printed in Great Britain by The Whitefriars Press Ltd
London and Tonbridge

## PREFACE

This is an attempt to present the essential facts of gynaecology in a book that can literally be carried in the pocket. There has been strict economy of words, not omission of facts. The present edition has been thoroughly revised, and new material is included.

S.G.C.

London, 1972

# CONTENTS

Chapter 1

# ANATOMY

### Vulva and Superficial Perineal Structures

The *labia majora* are two skin folds containing fatty tissue which bound the vulval cleft and meet anteriorly in the mons pubis. The labia and mons bear hair follicles and sebaceous glands. The *labia minora* are two narrow skin folds lying between the labia majora. The labia minora enclose the *vaginal vestibule,* and each divides anteriorly to form the prepuce of the clitoris. The *clitoris* consists of erectile tissue arranged in two corpora cavernosa and a glans, the latter having a rich nerve supply. The *superficial perineal muscles* are shown in the diagrams (Figs 1 and 2). Bulbo-cavernosus arises from the

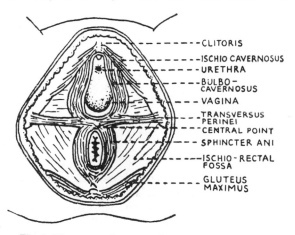

Fig. 1. Diagram to show superficial perineal muscles.

central point and is inserted into the corpus cavernosum. Ischio-cavernosus arises from the pubic ramus and is inserted into the crus clitoridis. Transversus perinei arises from the ischial tuberosity and is inserted into the central point. The *vestibular bulbs* of erectile tissue lie beneath the bulbo-cavernosus muscle on either side of the vaginal orifice. The *greater vestibular glands of Bartholin* lie immediately posterior to the vestibular bulbs, on either side, and are compound racemose glands, with cubical epithelium. The *perineal membrane* (triangular ligament) fills in the subpubic arch and

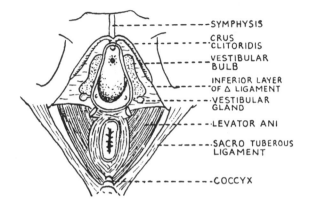

Fig. 2. Diagram to show superficial perineal structures after removal of superficial muscles.

has two layers, between which the compressor urethrae (deep transverse perineal) muscle lies. The *perineal body* occupies the space between the lowest third of the vagina and the anal canal, and consists of fibrous tissue with muscle fibres from levator ani and the perineal muscles.

## The Vagina

The vagina passes upwards and backwards, at a right angle to the axis of the uterus. The anterior wall is 7 cm long, and related to the urethra and bladder. The posterior wall is 9 cm long, and related in the lower third to the perineal body, in the middle third to the rectum, and in the upper third to the recto-vaginal pouch of peritoneum. The lumen is flattened so that the anterior and posterior walls are in contact. The cervix uteri projects into the vaginal vault to divide it into four *fornices.* The shallow anterior fornix is related to the bladder, and the deep posterior fornix to the recto-vaginal pouch. Each lateral fornix is related to the base of the broad ligament, which contains the ureter, and the tubes and ovaries can be palpated through the lateral fornices. The vagina has a wall of smooth muscle, and a rugose lining of squamous epithelium without glands. Oestrogen causes proliferation of the epithelial cells, which become more stratified and contain glycogen, which is the precursor of the lactic acid found in the vaginal secretion. In the virgin the vaginal orifice is partly closed by the hymeneal membrane.

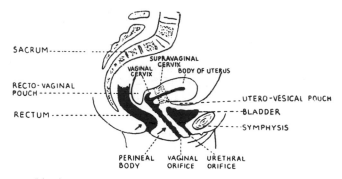

Fig. 3. Diagram of sagittal section of pelvis. (Arrows show direction of action of levator ani.)

## The Uterus

The uterus is pear-shaped, and 7.5 cm long with a cavity of 6 cm. It is divided into cervix (2.5 cm long) and body; the part of the body above the tubal orifices is the fundus. The fundus is directed forwards (*anteversion*) and the body is slightly bent forwards on the cervix (*anteflexion*).

**The Cervix** consists of the vaginal portion which projects into the vault, and the supravaginal portion above. The cervical canal is spindle shaped, and extends upwards from the external os to the internal os, where it is continuous with the uterine cavity. In nulliparae the external os is small and circular, but in parous women it is oval and often lacerated. The cervical canal has glands which branch deeply into the fibro-muscular wall of the cervix. The epithelium consists of tall columnar cells, with basal nuclei, and there is no interglandular stroma. Menstrual bleeding does not occur from it, although oestrogens cause the glands to secrete clear mucus, as seen at the mid-point of the menstrual cycle.

The cervix is not directly related to the peritoneum except on the posterior aspect of its supravaginal portion. Tumours arising from the cervix tend to extend into the base of the broad ligament where they may displace the ureter upwards.

**The Body of the Uterus** is covered with peritoneum, except for a narrow area on either side, where the broad ligaments are attached. The wall is 1 cm thick, and chiefly consists of smooth muscle, with less fibrous tissue than in the cervix. The uterine cavity is triangular, with the apex inferiorly at the

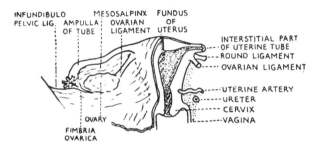

Fig. 4. Posterior view of broad ligament.

internal os, and a tubal opening at each upper angle. The endometrium has simple tubular glands of columnar epithelium set in a vascular stroma. Unlike those of the cervix, the glands do not penetrate into the muscle coat, and menstrual changes occur. (See p. 14.)

**Relations of the Uterus.** The uterus is freely mobile, and situated centrally in the pelvic cavity. Anteriorly the peritoneum of the utero-vesical pouch covers the uterine body down to the level of the internal os, and below that the supravaginal cervix is related to the base of the bladder. Posteriorly, the uterine body is covered with peritoneum, which is continued downwards over the supravaginal cervix and vaginal vault. Laterally the uterus is related to the broad ligaments, and the ureter passes forwards half an inch from the side of the cervix, with the uterine artery crossing above it.

### The Uterine (Fallopian) Tubes

The two tubes extent outwards from the uterine cornua,

and lie in the upper free edges of the broad ligaments. The part of the tube in the uterine wall is the interstitial portion, and is succeeded by the narrow isthmus, with a lumen of less than 1 mm in diameter. The tube then widens out as the ampulla, and curves round the ovary before opening into the peritoneal cavity at the abdominal ostium. The ostium is surrounded by fimbriae, and one fimbria is longer than the others and attached to the lower pole of the ovary (fimbria ovarica). The tube has a complete peritoneal coat, except below at the mesosalpinx, and a wall of smooth muscle. The mucosa is arranged in complex longitudinal folds, so that on section the lumen appears full of plicae. The epithelium bears cilia, which work towards the uterus.

## The Ovaries

Each ovary is about 3.5 cm long, and is attached to the back of the broad ligament. The surface of the ovary is wrinkled, and covered with a single layer of cubical cells (germinal epithelium), which is continuous with the peritoneal mesothelium at the hilum. The cortex contains the follicular elements scattered among the spindle-shaped stroma cells. The stroma is denser at the surface (tunica albuginea). The medulla is the small portion at the hilum containing vessels and embryonic rudiments (rete ovarii).

**Ovarian (Graafian) Follicles** are seen in various stages of ripeness (Fig. 5). The primitive follicle consists of a central large cell, surrounded by a single ring of cells. As the follicle ripens the cells around the ovum proliferate to become several layers deep, and are known as granulosa cells. As the granulosa cells increase in number, a space containing fluid appears, and then splits them into a smaller mass of cells surrounding the ovum (discus proligerus) and a larger sheet of cells that line the follicle. Outside the granulosa cells is a layer of smaller theca-interna cells, and outside these the stroma is condensed to form the theca externa. The ripe ovum is about 0.1 mm in diameter with an eccentric nucleus and nucleolus.

At birth the ovary contains thousands of follicles, but only one ripens fully in each normal menstrual cycle. This follicle approaches the surface of the ovary as it enlarges, and at ovulation the ovum and a few surrounding granulosa cells are discharged into the peritoneal cavity. After ovulation the follicle becomes the *corpus luteum.* The granulosa cells lining the follicle accumulate lipoid and are now called lutein cells,

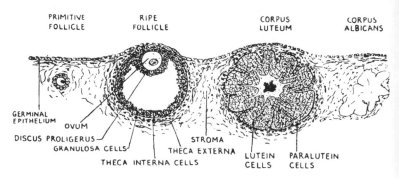

Fig. 5. Diagram of Graafian follicle and corpus luteum.

and a similar change occurs in the theca-interna cells, which are now called paralutein cells. Both layers become infolded into the empty cavity of the follicle. When the corpus luteum finally degenerates, it shrinks to a hyaline mass, the *corpus albicans.*

## The Broad Ligaments

The broad ligaments are two transverse peritoneal folds which extend outwards from the lateral borders of the uterus to the pelvic wall on either side. (See Fig. 4.) The upper free edge encloses the uterine tube, and this part of the ligament is termed the *mesosalpinx.* Beyond the tubal ostium the broad ligament is continued outwards to the pelvic wall as the *infundibulo-pelvic ligament.* The ovary is attached to the back of the broad ligament, and the ovarian vessels and nerves pass between its layers. The base of the broad ligament widens out, so that the two peritoneal sheets of which it is composed are further apart, leaving a space containing loose cellular tissue, in which the uterine vessels and nerves and the ureter lie. Wolffian rudiments found in the broad ligament are described on p. 21.

## The Ovarian Ligaments and the Round Ligaments

The *ovarian ligament* extends from the ovary to the uterine cornu, and then continues forwards (below the tube) as the *round ligament of the uterus*. The round ligament runs beneath the peritoneum to the deep abdominal ring, and passes down the inguinal canal to end in the labium majus. Both ligaments contain smooth muscle fibres and together they correspond to the gubernaculum of the testis.

## The Pelvic Cellular Tissue

The spaces between the pelvic organs, and especially between the layers of the broad ligaments in their wider basal parts, are filled with loose cellular tissue, which is continuous with the extraperitoneal tissue of the anterior and posterior abdominal walls, and also with extrapelvic fasciae through the various pelvic foramina. Infection can spread by all these routes. Certain denser bands are described separately below, but these supporting bands are part of the pelvic cellular tissue. The main mass of cellular tissue at the side of the uterus is known as the *parametrium*.

## The Supports of the Uterus

It is strongly emphasized that the broad ligaments are only peritoneal folds, and that the direction of the round ligaments is such that they cannot support the uterus but only maintain it in anteversion. The real supports of the uterus are the cardinal and utero-sacral ligaments. Each *cardinal ligament* (transverse pelvic ligament) extends from the side wall of the pelvis near the white line to the supravaginal cervix and vaginal fault. It is a fan-shaped sheet of fibro-muscular tissue, almost continuous behind the utero-sacral ligament. The ureter runs forward between the upper fibres of the ligament. The *utero-sacral ligaments* pass from the cervix to the sacrum. The rectum and recto-vaginal peritoneal pouch lie between them. (Fig. 6.)

These ligaments are part of the visceral pelvic fascia, which also gives rise to tubular investments of the vagina and rectum. A condensation of the fascia beneath the bladder is sometimes described as the *pubo-cervical ligament* but does not compare for density and strength with the other ligaments.

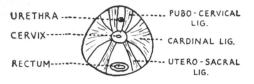

Fig. 6. Diagram of pelvis (from above) to show
pelvic ligaments.

## The Supports of the Vagina. The Pelvic Floor

The anterior and posterior vaginal walls are in contact, and anything that supports the posterior wall will therefore indirectly support the anterior wall and the bladder. The lowest third of the posterior wall is related to the perineal body, into which levator ani and the superficial perineal muscle are inserted. The *levator ani muscle* arises from the pubic bone, from the white line (arcus tendineus) over obturator internus, and from the ischial spine. The fibres pass backwards, downwards and inwards to be inserted into the perineal body, the anal canal, and the ano-coccygeal raphé. With its fellow of the opposite side levator ani forms a sling which draws the perineal body forwards and upwards, and so supports the vaginal walls and bladder. The urethra and vagina pass forwards between the medial edges of the levator muscles, and some of the muscle fibres are inserted into them.

## Blood Supply of the Pelvic Organs

The *ovarian artery* is a branch of the abdominal aorta. After crossing the pelvic brim it passes medially in the infundibulo-pelvic ligament and divides into branches that supply ovary, tube and the upper part of the uterus. The left *ovarian vein* joins the renal vein, the right enters the inferior vena cava.

The *uterine artery* is a branch of the hypogastric (internal iliac) artery. It passes medially in the base of the broad ligament, where the ureter runs forward beneath it. Before reaching the uterus cervical and vaginal branches are given off, and in the uterine wall branches arise which encircle the uterus to anastomose with branches from the opposite side, and also with the ovarian artery. A separate vaginal artery may arise from the hypogastric artery. The *uterine veins* drain into the hypogastric veins.

The *pudendal artery,* which also arises from the hypogastric artery, runs forward on the lateral wall of the ischio-rectal fossa, and gives off inferior haemorrhoidal and perineal branches. The *perineal veins* drain into the pudic veins, but the *dorsal vein of the clitoris* drains directly backwards into the vesical plexus.

## Lymphatic Drainage of the Pelvic Organs

Lymphatic vessels from the upper part of the body of the uterus, and from the tubes and ovaries, drain upwards to the pre-aortic glands. A few vessels sometimes accompany the round ligament and drain into the inguinal glands.

Lymphatics from the lower part of the body of the uterus, the cervix and the upper two-thirds of the vagina, drain into the iliac and obdurator glands. A few vessels run backwards with the uterosacral ligaments to the sacral glands.

Lymphatics from the lower third of the vagina and the vulva drain into the inguinal glands.

## Nerve Supply of the Pelvic Organs

**Perineal Structures.** The pudendal nerve gives sensory and motor branches to the perineum. The ilio-inguinal nerve gives sensory branches to the labium majus.

**Viscera.** *Efferent nerves:* The orthosympathetic outflow from the lower dorsal and upper two lumbar spinal segments gives fibres which ultimately reach the pre-aortic plexus. This is continued downwards as the superior hypogastric plexus ('presacral nerve'), which lies in the retroperitoneal tissue in front of the last lumbar vertebra. This plexus bifurcates to form the right and left inferior hypogastric plexuses, which are joined by parasympathetic fibres from the second, third and fourth sacral nerves. The fibres run forward with the utero-sacral ligaments to the pelvic plexuses and ganglia (of

Frankenhäuser) in the parametrium, and then supply the uterus and bladder. The parasympathetic element is probably excitor to the main uterine musculature and inhibitor to the cervical muscle, and the orthosympathetic element has the opposite action.

*Afferent nerves:* Afferent nerves from the uterus follow the same pathways in reverse, but there is an additional afferent path. Fibres from the ovary, tube and uterine fundus accompany the ovarian vessels, and pass upwards to the renal plexus, finally reaching the posterior roots of the tenth, eleventh and twelfth dorsal and first lumbar segments. (We have no knowledge of efferent fibres in the ovarian plexus.)

## Chapter 2

# PHYSIOLOGY OF THE REPRODUCTIVE SYSTEM

The whole reproductive system is controlled by hormones from the pituitary gland, assisted by placental hormones during pregnancy.

## The Hypothalamus

In many animals the hypothalamus can be shown to control pituitary gonadotrophic function by the secretion of humoral factors which pass along the veins in the pituitary stalk to reach the gland. The release factor for gonadotrophin has been shown to be a decapeptide which has been synthesized. It is not yet available for therapy. Stimuli from the cerebral cortex affect hypothalamic function.

## Anterior Pituitary Gonadotrophic Hormones

At about the age of 11 hypothalamic activity starts to stimulate the basophil cells of the anterior pituitary to secrete gonadotrophic hormones which control ovulation and the secretion of ovarian hormones. In a normal cycle ovulation only occurs once, 12-14 days after the onset of the preceding period.

There are two pituitary gonadotrophins, both glyco-proteins. *Follicle Stimulating Hormone* (FSH) causes ripening of the ovarian follicle (p. 5). The level of FSH rises from the first to the 10th day of the cycle and then falls. *Luteinizing Hormone* (LH)—sometimes called Interstitial Cell Stimulating Hormone (ICSH)—is constantly present, but in increased amount from the 12th to the 14th day of cycle. Ovulation occurs at a critical point when the concentration of FSH is falling and that of LH is rising. After ovulation LH causes accumulation of cholesterol-like substances in the granulosa and theca interna cells (see corpus luteum, p. 6).

The view that a third hormone (prolactin, luteotrophin) is also necessary for maintenance of the human corpus luteum is not now generally held.

In response to gonadotrophins the ripening follicle secretes oestrogens, and after ovulation the corpus luteum secretes both oestrogens and progesterone. Oestrogens inhibit the output of FSH; this check occurs in each cycle. It is believed, with less certainty, that progesterone inhibits the output of LH. After the menopause, when ovarian activity ceases, the output of gonadotrophins is increased for a time.

Gonadotrophins are excreted in the urine, where they can be measured by radioimmunoassay. (See also p. 115.)

## The Ovarian Hormones

These hormones are produced by the ovarian follicle and corpus luteum in response to pituitary gonadotrophins.

**Oestrogens.** There are several oestrogenic steroids. That secreted by the ovary is oestradiol, and this is partly converted to less active oestrone and oestriol and also conjugated with glucuronic acid before being excreted in the urine. Only 10 per cent of the ovarian output appears in the urine; the rest is fixed by the endometrium or inactivated by the liver. The total urinary output is about 1 mg per month, and the maximum urinary output (at mid-cycle) is about 100 $\mu$g per 24 hours.

The specific effects of oestrogens are:

VULVA: Increased vascularity and enlargement of labia.

VAGINA: Epithelial proliferation with cornification and accumulation of glycogen in cells.

CERVIX: Secretion of clear mucus.

UTERINE AND TUBAL MUSCLE: Hypertrophy and increased contractility.

ENDOMETRIUM: Increased vascularity and proliferation of both glands and stroma. (Oestrogens acting intermittently, as in menstrual cycles, produce normal proliferation, but if oestrogens act continuously for several weeks pathological hyperplasia occurs.)

SECONDARY SEXUAL CHARACTERISTICS: Growth of pubic and axillary hair, feminine fat distribution, feminine libido and psyche.

BREASTS: Duct proliferation.

ANTERIOR PITUITARY GLAND: Inhibition of the production of FSH and growth hormone.

The chemistry is described on p. 115 and synthetic oestrogens on p. 117.

**Progesterone**. Progesterone is the precursor in the body of corticosteroids, androgens and oestrogens, and there is a low but constant level in the blood. In addition about 300 mg are secreted in each cycle by the corpus luteum, so that the blood level rises after ovulation. A proportion of this is secreted in the urine as biologically inert pregnanediol glucuronide, which can be estimated chemically. The maximum daily output of pregnanediol in the third week of the cycle is about 5 mg per 24 hours.

The specific effects of progesterone are:

VAGINA: The epithelial cells show further changes which can be recognized in a smear. The cells become more basophil and more clumped together.

CERVICAL MUCUS: If mid-cycle mucus is dried on a slide it forms a fern-like pattern of salt crystals. Later in the cycle this does not occur if ovulation has taken place.

ENDOMETRIUM: If previously 'primed' by oestrogens secretory change and decidual reaction occur (p. 14).

UTERINE AND TUBAL MUSCLE: In some species motility is decreased, but in women stronger, though slower, contractions occur.

BREASTS: If previous duct proliferation has been induced by oestrogens, proliferation of acini follows.

ANTERIOR PITUITARY GLAND: Present knowledge suggests that progesterone inhibits the production of LH.

TEMPERATURE: After ovulation the basal temperature rises $0.5°C$.

The chemistry is described on p. 115 and synthetic progestogens on p. 118.

**Androgens**. Even in normal women some androgens are secreted by the suprarenal cortex and excreted in the urine. They appear to have little physiological effect in health.

## The Menstrual Cycle (Fig. 7)

For convenience the normal adult function is described before the changes that occur at puberty.

During the first half of the menstrual cycle the ripening follicle secretes oestrogens, and the blood level rises steadily, except that a transitory fall may occur at the time of ovulation. During the second half of the cycle the corpus luteum secretes both oestrogens and progesterone, and the blood level of both hormones reaches a peak a few days before menstruation is due. If the ovum liberated in that cycle is not fertilized there is a fall in the level of both hormones and menstruation occurs.

Immediately after menstruation the uterus is lined by a simple cubical epithelium, with short tubular glands and scanty interglandular stroma. Under the influence of oestrogens the endometrium becomes more vascular, and the tubular glands longer, with columnar cells. After ovulation, when the action of progesterone is added, the glands secrete mucus, so that each gland becomes distended and has a crenated outline. The stromal cells swell and are now called decidual cells, and the stroma becomes more compact, especially near the surface. If a fertilized ovum embeds in the endometrium this decidual reaction persists, otherwise menstruation occurs and the endometrium breaks down. This disintegration is due to ischaemic necrosis, as the endometrial arterioles contract and cut off the blood supply to all but the deepest layer. The mucoid contents of the glands are discharged together with blood and endometrial fragments, the uterus contracting actively. After menstruation regeneration of the endometrium takes place from the residual basal layer.

The precise cause of menstruation is still uncertain. The arterial spasm is an acetyl-choline effect which can be precipitated by injections of prostigmine in the premenstrual phase. Probably the withdrawal of oestrogens is the chief factor, although withdrawal of progesterone may play some part.

Ovarian hormones inhibit the production of gonadotrophins and each cycle may be likened to a see-saw; first the pituitary hormones stimulate the ovary, then the ovarian hormones inhibit the pituitary. Apart from the 'automatic'

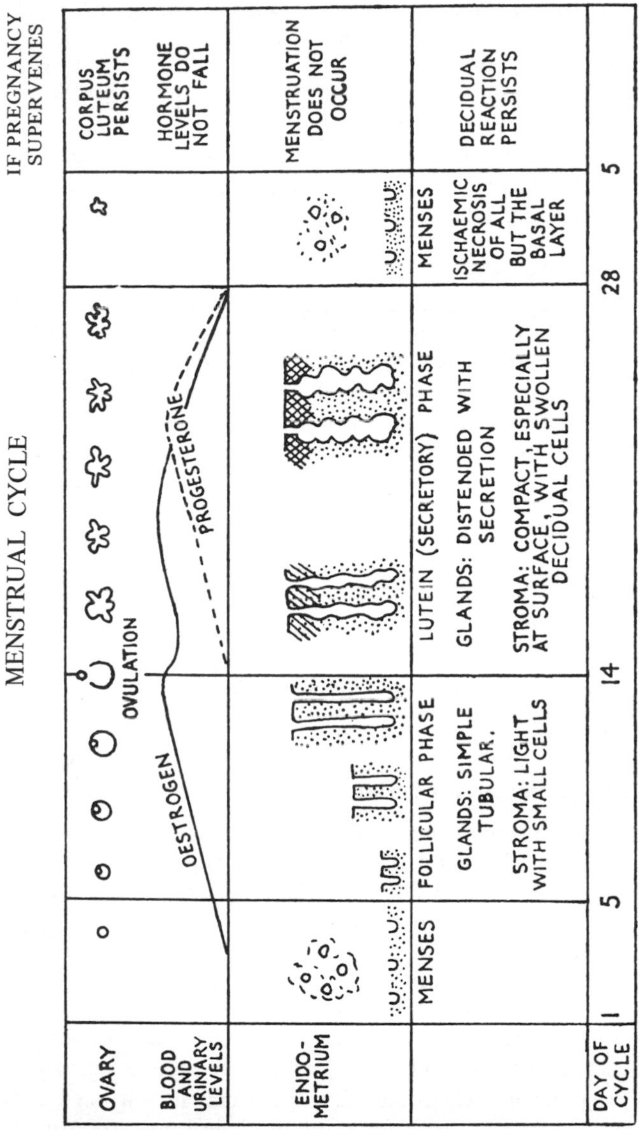

MENSTRUAL CYCLE

IF PREGNANCY SUPERVENES

| OVARY | | | | | | CORPUS LUTEUM PERSISTS |
|---|---|---|---|---|---|---|
| BLOOD AND URINARY LEVELS | OESTROGEN | OVULATION | PROGESTERONE | | | HORMONE LEVELS DO NOT FALL |
| ENDO-METRIUM | MENSES | FOLLICULAR PHASE<br>GLANDS: SIMPLE TUBULAR.<br>STROMA: LIGHT WITH SMALL CELLS | LUTEIN (SECRETORY) PHASE<br>GLANDS: DISTENDED WITH SECRETION<br>STROMA: COMPACT, ESPECIALLY AT SURFACE, WITH SWOLLEN DECIDUAL CELLS | | MENSES<br>ISCHAEMIC NECROSIS OF ALL BUT THE BASAL LAYER | MENSTRUATION DOES NOT OCCUR<br><br>DECIDUAL REACTION PERSISTS |
| DAY OF CYCLE | 1 | 5 | 14 | 28 | 5 | |

Fig. 7. Physiology of the reproductive system.

endocrine control, emotion such as fear, or sexual stimuli, may alter the rhythm, presumably by nervous stimuli acting on the hypothalamus, and so in turn on the pituitary gland.

The normal cycle is of 28 days including five days of menstruation; but cycles of from 21 to 35 days, with three to seven days of menstruation are within normal limits. The discharge over a whole period measures 30-150 ml, but only half of this is blood; mucus predominates in early and late stages. Clots are unusual as they are liquefied by endometrial ferments unless the bleeding is too heavy for this to occur. Many healthy women have symptoms such as emotional tension or depression, lassitude, headache, pelvic discomfort and slight frequency just before or during menstruation; but severe or incapacitating pain must be regarded as abnormal. Slight breast enlargement and discomfort are common. Psychological factors certainly accentuate menstrual complaints, but there is objective evidence of metabolic changes; for example, temperature changes, and gain of weight due to retention of water and sodium chloride. The term *premenstrual tension* is used for such symptoms. It is claimed that these can be relieved by giving 1 g capsules of ammonium chloride thrice daily in the premenstrual week, or by giving oral progestogens, such as oral norethisterone 20 mg daily from the 15th to the 25th day of the cycle, but sedatives and tranquillizers, such as meprobamate 200 mg thrice daily, are probably just as effective.

### Early Pregnancy. Chorionic Gonadotrophic Hormone

If a fertilized ovum embeds in the endometrium, the chorionic trophoblast of the ovum produces chorionic gonadotrophin. This differs from the pituitary gonadotrophins described above (e.g., it has no action on the hypophysectomized animal). It is excreted in the urine, and diagnostic pregnancy tests such as the biological Hogben and Aschheim-Zondek tests and the immunological tests depend on its detection there. During pregnancy the corpus luteum persists, because of this hormone, and continues to secrete oestrogens and progesterone which maintain the decidua. In women after the first 10 weeks the corpus luteum is not essential for the maintenance of pregnancy, as both progesterone and oestrogens are directly produced by the placenta.

## The Lower Genital Tract

The normal thick white vaginal secretion is highly acid ($p$H 4). In response to oestrogens, the stratified cells accumulate glycogen, which is converted to lactic acid by Döderlein's bacilli, which are constantly present. The acidity is a barrier against ascending infection, but quickly kills spermatozoa.

The cervical glands secrete an alkaline mucus, which alters in different phases of the menstrual cycle. At mid-cycle the mucus is less viscous, and spermatozoa can more easily enter it to gain protection from the vaginal acid. Semen contains hyaluronidase, a ferment that liquefies cervical mucus. Sexual stimulation increases cervical secretion and so may make fertilization more probable, and both cervical and vestibular mucus has a lubricating function in coitus.

Cyclical changes in the cells of the vaginal epithelium can be shown by staining smears of the desquamated cells.

## Puberty

We now return to consider the events that occur before menstruation starts. Gonadotrophins are secreted from the age of about 11, but the ovary only responds at a certain maturity. The first response is the production of oestrogens; ovulation may not always occur in early cycles.

Puberty usually occurs between 12 and 15 years. The whole configuration of the body alters. Skeletal growth slows, female characteristics of the pelvis are accentuated, subcutaneous fat becomes of adult distribution, and the breasts enlarge. Pubic hair appears and the labia majora become larger. The body of the uterus enlarges and now becomes longer than the cervix. Menstruation starts, and other endocrine changes occur, especially thyroid enlargement and shrinkage of the thymus.

Delayed puberty may be of serious import. One-third of women who do not menstruate before the age of 17 have permanent amenorrhoea. Such delay is theoretically due to hypothalamic dysfunction, pituitary deficiency, ovarian dysgensis (p. 26), failure of uterine response or vaginal atresia; but any disorder of general health or nutrition may indirectly affect the reproductive cycle.

Excessive bleeding may occur in early cycles, as a result of unbalanced production of oestrogens (see p. 91).

Very rarely precocious uterine bleeding is due to oestrogens from a granulosa cell tumour, but in most cases of early puberty ovarian uterine function and structure are normal. These 'constitutional' cases do not require treatment.

## The Menopause

Endocrine changes at the end of the reproductive period are almost the reverse of those at puberty. The ovarian response ceases, first by failure of ovulation so that progesterone is no longer produced by the ovary, and eventually all ovarian oestrogenic activity ceases. For a time the output of gonadotrophins increases, but finally that too diminishes. The thyroid becomes less active, and sometimes the suprarenal cortex more active.

The ovaries atrophy, and the uterus shrinks to a length of about 2 cm, the vaginal portion becoming especially shortened so as to become flush with the vault. The muscle is largely replaced by fibrous tissue, and the endometrium becomes a thin layer with scanty glands. The vagina narrows and vaginal actidity falls; the labia shrink and pubic hair is lost.

The cessation of menstruation is termed the menopause and usually occurs between 45 and 50 years, though sometimes earlier or later. The commonest event is a gradual increase in the interval between periods, with diminishing loss at each successive period; but sometimes menstruation ceases abruptly. Although common, any *excessive or irregular loss must be regarded as pathological* and investigated. Depression and emotional instability are common, libido may be reduced, but is not usually completely lost. 'Hot flushes' (intermittent vasodilatation of face and trunk) may occur, due to the temporary high level of gonadotrophins. Weight is often gained as thyroid activity diminishes.

These symptoms may be accepted as 'normal', but more severe degenerative changes in the vulva (p. 43), or ascending infection due to the low vaginal acidity (p. 46) are regarded as pathological. Though certain other disorders occur in women of menopausal age (e.g., hypertension, osteoarthritis, and involutional psychoses) they are probably unrelated to the changes in the reproductive hormones. True menopausal symptoms such as 'hot flushes' and vaginal changes respond to oestrogens. Start with stilboestrol 0.5 mg daily by mouth, and reduce the dose as soon as possible, otherwise bleeding may be induced. Alternatively a combination of oestrogens and androgens may be used, e.g. 5 mg methyltestosterone with 0.01 mg ethinyl oestradiol.

Chapter 3

# EMBRYOLOGY AND CONGENITAL ABNORMALITIES

## The External Genitalia and Urogenital Sinus

The diagram (Fig. 8) shows the tail end of an early embryo. Allantois and hind-gut open into the cloaca, which is subdivided into urogenital sinus and rectum by the down-growth of the septum (S). The two passages are for a time obscured by the cloacal membrane, but when this disappears two separate openings are seen. In front of the cloaca, the genital tubecle gives rise to the clitoris, and lateral folds pass back from it on each side to form the labia.

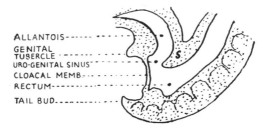

Fig. 8. Diagram of sagittal section of hind-end of embryo.

The allantois, which forms the upper part of the bladder, opens into the urogenital sinus; and the urogenital sinus forms the bladder base, urethra and vestibule. The Müllerian ducts grow downwards in the septum (S) between the urogenital sinus and blind-gut, and thus the genital tract comes to lie between the urinary tract and rectum.

## The Ovary

In the early embryo, the gonad appears on the posterior wall of the coelom as a longitudinal ridge of mesoderm. The covering epithelium becomes the germinal epithelium, so-called as it was formerly believed that ova developed from it.

It is now known that primitive sex cells migrate into the gonad from the wall of the yolk-sac.

The genital ridge is continued downwards to the inguinal region, and a gubernaculum appears in it. The ovary descends from its primitive lumbar position, and the gubernaculum persists as the ovarian and uterine round ligaments.

### The Uterine Tube, Uterus and Vagina

A second ridge appears laterally to the ovary, and in this the Müllerian and Wolffian ducts appear. The cephalic end of the Müllerian duct opens into the coelom at the future site of the tubal ostium. The caudal parts of the two Müllerian ducts fuse in the midline, and then grow downwards as a solid core of cells in the septum between the urogenital sinus and rectum, finally joining the urogenital sinus low down on its posterior wall. It was formerly taught that this core became canalized to form the vagina, the hymen marking the site of the original opening into the urogenital sinus, but more recent work suggests that the vaginal epithelium grows upwards from the urogenital sinus to the cervix.

The mesoderm surrounding the Müllerian epithelium gives rise to muscle fibres. The unfused upper ducts become the uterine tubes and the fused ducts below give rise to the uterus and vagina.

### Wolffian Structures (Fig. 9)

In the female, the Wolffian duct system becomes vestigial, except for the part which forms the ureter. The Wolffian duct

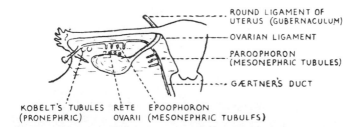

Fig. 9. Diagram to show Wolffian structures.

appears as a longitudinal duct, parallel to the Müllerian duct, and a series of tubules open into it: (1) At the cephalic end pronephric tubules representing the most primitive excretory system appear, and may persist as small Kobelt's tubules in the outer mesosalpinx, often becoming pedunculated. (2) Mesonephric tubules appear beside the intermediate part of the duct, and some of these become the excretory duct of the gonad in the male. Even in the female a transitory system of junctional tubules (the rete ovarii) unite these ducts and the gonad. Epoöphoric and paroöphoric tubules, which may give rise to small cysts, are sometimes found in the mesosalpinx and represent mesonephric tubules. Remains of the rete ovarii may be found in the hilum of the ovary.

The Wolffian duct itself may persist, running beside the uterus and vagina, where it is named Gaertner's duct, and may give rise to lateral vaginal cysts.

# CONGENITAL ABNORMALITIES

## The Ovaries

The ovary may only be represented by a fibrous 'streak' in cases of gonadal dysgenesis (p. 26) resulting from chromosomal abnormality. There is primary amenorrhoea. No treatment is possible.

## Wolffian Vestiges

Described above, and of little clinical importance.

## The Uterine Tubes

If the uterus is rudimentary, both tubes may be absent, and with malformation of half of the uterus the corresponding tube may be rudimentary. Accessory abdominal ostia and diverticula occur; the latter may be the site of an ectopic pregnancy.

## The Uterus. Arrest of Development of the Whole Uterus

(1) The rudimentary uterus only consists of a nodule of fibrous tissue. Function is absent and treatment hopeless.

(2) The infantile uterus corresponds in form with that of the child at birth, and the cervix is relatively much longer than in the adult. There is usually primary amenorrhoea. Treatment with oestrogens may be attempted but seldom succeeds.

**Imperfect Müllerian Fusion**. The varying degrees of this condition are best described by illustration (Fig. 10).

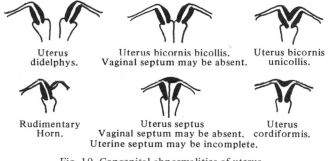

Fig. 10. Congenital abnormalities of uterus.

These abnormalities may cause surprisingly little functional disturbance. If pregnancy occurs in one horn the other empty horn shows hypertrophy and decidual development. In exceptional cases abortion may occur, or obstruction in labour may arise from malpresentation, or because the non-pregnant horn lies below the presenting part.

In the case of a rudimentary horn, pregnancy is more dangerous, as the horn ruptures with intraperitoneal bleeding. The symptoms resemble those of tubal ectopic pregnancy (p. 107), except that the accident occurs later (often at the 16th week). The treatment is laparotomy and excision of the horn.

**Congenital Elongation of the Cervix**. In this condition the cervix may extend down to the vaginal orifice. The fornices are of normal depth, in contrast to the shallow fornices in cases of prolapse. If there is dyspareunia the redundant cervix is amputated.

### The Vagina

*Vaginal septa* have already been mentioned. Imperfect

Müllerian canalization may occur so that the vagina is absent, or show atresia of varying extent. The commonest site of obstruction is just above the hymen, usually by a thin membrane. If the vagina is imperforate and uterine function is normal, menstrual secretion accumulates in the vagina and distends it, a condition called *haematocolpos*. The haematocolpos may be large enough to be palpable from the abdomen, and to form a pelvic tumour which displaces the bladder upwards and causes urinary retention. The other symptoms are amenorrhoea, with pain at monthly intervals, noticed a few months after the expected onset of puberty. The occluding membrane is seen bulging, and is bluish in colour if retained blood is seen through it. The treatment is to excise the membrane. The tarry contents should not be douched away as there is a risk of ascending infection but merely absorbed on sterile pads.

In cases of *absent vagina,* treatment may be sought to allow normal intercourse. In McIndoe's operation a cavity is dissected at the site of the vagina, and a suitable mould carrying a Thiersch graft is inserted and stitched in place for several weeks to prevent contraction of the cavity. In Williams's operation, which is rather simpler, the posterior parts of the labia minora are sutured together to form a tubular recess.

## Abnormalities of the Urinary Tract

In cases of congenital abnormalities of the uterus or vagina intravenous pyelographs often show urinary abnormalities such as double ureter, or absence of the kidney on one side.

## Sexual Determination

In cases of abnormal anatomical development the determination of sex may be extremely difficult, and even the scientific definition of 'sex' is not easy. It has hitherto been usual to define the sex by the type of gonad present, but uncertainties arise when the gonads are of mixed type or undifferentiated, and the configuration of the body and the form of the external genital organs (phenotype) may not correspond to the sex of the gonads. Even in individuals of normal physical development difficulties of psychology and behaviour may arise.

It has recently been shown that the basic sexual differentiation is determined by the genes, which are parts of the nuclear chromosomes. There are normally 46 chromosomes in each cell of the human body. In the reduction division during maturation of the sex cells these chromosomes divide into 23 pairs, so that each ovum or sperm contains half the ordinary complement. The majority of the chromosomes (the autosomes) divide into pairs that appear identical, but two of the chromosomes (the sex chromosomes) show specialization. In the female the sex chromosomes consist of paired XX chromosomes, so that after the reduction division every ovum contains an X chromosome. In the male the sex chromosomes consist of an X chromosome and a smaller Y chromosome, so that after the reduction division some sperms will contain an X chromosome and some a Y chromosome. Conjugation of sperms and ova give rise to XX and XY pairs again, as shown in the scheme:

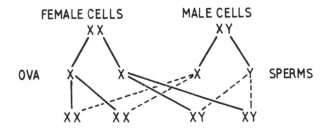

Every normal body cell has this male or female constitution, and this is the basis of the determination of 'nuclear sex'. Cells which contain two XX chromosomes have a nodule of chromatin which can be seen with the microscope, and which distinguishes such cells from XY cells, or from abnormal cells which contain only one X chromosome. (Abnormal cells with more than two X chromosomes may have more than one visible chromatin nodule.) The test is usually made on polymorphonuclear leukocytes or cells scraped from buccal epithelium. It should be realized that it is the invisible genes which determine sex, and these are not only found in the sex chromosomes but are scattered among the autosomes; yet the visible chromosomal pattern is a useful laboratory test that gives at least a partial indication of the genetic pattern.

In normal females the combined influence of the genes of the paired XX chromosomes and of the autosomes causes development of the cortex of the gonad to form an ovary, and the development of the Müllerian system. In normal males, with XY chromosomes, the genes (chiefly those of the autosomes) cause suppression of the development of the cortex of the gonad and the medulla develops into a testis, while the Wolffian system predominates. The development of the gonad seems to be determined by the primitive germ cells that migrate into it from the region of the yolk-sac in early embryonic life. The gonad ultimately establishes a male or female hormonal pattern, which causes the sexual changes of puberty.

## Abnormal Sexual Differentiation and Intersex

The ill-defined term *intersex* is applied to patients in whom the diagnosis of sex is difficult. Some have genetic (chromosomal) abnormalities, some have hormonal disorders, and in some there are developmental errors such as hypospadias with undescended testes. Abnormal psychological orientation is not usually due to chromosomal or hormonal effects.

**Gonadal Dysgenesis.** This term is applied to patients with female phenotype in whom the gonads are only represented by fibrous streaks. Those with *Turner's Syndrome* are of short stature and may have associated congenital abnormalities, including coarctation of the aorta, a web-like skin fold on each side of the neck, and cubitus valgus. Most of these individuals have 45 chromosomes, and the nuclei do not have the nodule that indicates an XX pattern; it is probable that there has been an abnormal reduction division and that one X chromosome is missing.

Other patients with female phenotype and normal stature do not have the deformities of Turner's syndrome, and have a normal chromosomal pattern 46 XX. The reason for the failure of development of the gonads is unknown.

In *'Simple Dysgenesis'* the patients are tall, with primary amenorrhoea and failure of breast development, but have pubic and axillary hair. The chromosomal structure is 46 XY, and it is assumed that the Y chromosome is defective.

It is to be noted that absence of breast development with a female phenotype is indicative of gonadal dysgenesis.

**Klinefelter's Syndrome** only concerns the gynaecologist in the course of investigating infertility. The body form is male, with small but normal external genitals, but usually azoospermia. These individuals have 47 chromosomes, and the nuclear nodule is present; the structure is usually XXY.

**True Hermaphroditism** is exceedingly rare, but cases have been described with a testis on one side and an ovary on the other, with predominant development of the Müllerian and Wolffian tracts on the corresponding sides. There may be other abnormalities and the patients are usually infertile. The chromatin pattern may be of either type or a mosaic.

**Pseudohermaphroditism.** This term, perhaps more confusing than helpful, is applied to cases in which the outward sexual form differs from that of the gonads. One form of male pseudohermaphroditism is *Testicular Feminization,* in which the body form is female, with well-formed breasts and with pubic hair, but amenorrhoea is present, and the patient is found to have testes instead of ovaries. The chromatin pattern is that of a normal male. Testosterone is present in normal amounts, but for unknown reasons the tissues do not respond to it. The disorder may be familial. As there is a risk of disgerminoma (p. 75) arising, the gonads are removed after puberty.

Female pseudohermaphroditism has arisen in rare instances by masculinization of a female fetus by administration of large quantities of steroids, such as testosterone or progesterone, to the mother during pregnancy. Excessive secretion of androgens also occurs in the *Adrenogenital Syndrome.* This is a familial defect of function in which the suprarenal cortex fails to form hydrocortisone normally. Hydrocortisone normally inhibits the production of adrenocortical hormone by the pituitary gland, but in this disease the output of ACTH is unchecked, so that the abnormal suprarenal cortex is overstimulated, and it responds by the excessive production of androgens (it is unable to respond by producing hydrocortisone as a normal gland would). A female child may have a large clitoris and a cloaçal membrane so that the external organs resemble those of the male, although the internal organs are normal. The androgens cause masculinizing effects, and are excreted in the urine as oxosteroids which can be estimated. At a later stage there is amenorrhoea, hirsutes and excessive muscularity. The condition is sometimes reversible by giving cortisone, which inhibits the excessive output of ACTH.

**Management of Cases of Intersex**. In a child full investigation is essential, including nuclear sexing, oxosteroid and other hormonal estimations, pelvic examination under anaesthesia, and occasionally laparoscopy. Diagnostic problems include that of the male child with hypospadias and undescended testes. It is important that a child be brought up in the correct sex, and treatment is occasionally possible, e.g. for adrenogenital disorders, or by surgical modification of anatomical abnormalities. Oestrogens may cause breast development. In general the body form will determine the way an individual is brought up, and in older patients there is little purpose in altering the patient's mode of life, whatever the 'scientific' sex may be. Psychological problems, such as homosexuality (which usually has no relation to anatomical or hormonal abnormalities) are not considered here.

Chapter 4

# PELVIC INJURIES AND DISPLACEMENTS

Most gynaecological injuries follow childbirth, and prevention and immediate treatment is the duty of the obstetrician.

## Vulval and Perineal Injuries

Direct injury may cause lacerations or a haematoma. The latter may become large and painful and require incision to expel clot. If the bleeding point cannot be seen the cavity is packed with gauze. Very rarely a hymeneal tear may bleed enough to need suture.

If obstetrical tears of third degree involving the rectal sphincter are neglected, or break down from sepsis, they cause distressing incontinence for flatus or loose faeces. The perineal body is deficient, with the ends of the sphincter widely retracted, and the rectal mucosa exposed. Repair is delayed until all sepsis has subsided (p. 123).

## Vaginal Injuries

Apart from rare injuries at coitus, or in procuring abortion, these nearly always follow childbirth. *Prolapse* is described later for convenience (p. 32).

**Vesicovaginal Fistulae** may be due to (1) obstetrical injury, (2) operative injury, (3) radium burns, (4) ulceration of a neoplasm, usually cervical. Obstetrical injury may be immediate, by unskilful use of instruments, or delayed, when sloughing follows pressure in unduly prolonged labour. Operative injuries may occur at hysterectomy or colporrhaphy. (Radium burns and malignant fistulae are not considered further in this section.)

Vesicovaginal fistulae cause incontinence which is usually complete, but may be partial with small fistulae. The deep red bladder mucosa can be seen through a large opening, but small fistulae may only be found on cystoscopy or by injecting methylene blue into the nladder. Fistulae are often complicated by extensive scarring and by secondary cystitis and vulvovaginitis. Most traumatic fistulae can be closed by a vaginal operation. The vesical mucosa and vaginal skin are freed and sutured separately. Afterwards the bladder is kept drained with an in-dwelling catheter. In a difficult case a suprapubic cystotomy may be required, or an abdominal approach to the fistula. In the operation of colpocleisis the vaginal walls are sewn together below the fistula.

**Rectovaginal Fistulae** usually follow childbirth, but may also be due to neoplasm or radium burns. Recent obstetrical fistulae sometimes heal spontaneously; otherwise they are repaired by freeing the rectal mucosa and vaginal skin and suturing them separately.

**Ureteric Fistulae.** The ureter may be cut or tied during pelvic operations, or it may slough because of impaired blood supply after Wertheim's hysterectomy. Half the output of urine passes into the vaginal vault through the fistula. A pyelograph shows a dilated ureter above the fistula. Repair is seldom possible, and reimplantation into the bladder is usually required. Renal atrophy may occur if ureteric obstruction is unrelieved.

## Cervical Injuries

Minor cervical tears occur in every labour, but severe tears expose the cervical mucosa (ectropion), and the exposed mucosa gives rise to discharge. Such tears require repair (trachelorrhaphy, p. 121). Incompetence of the cervix, as a result of tears involving the internal os, or damage by injudicious surgical dilatation, may be a cause of miscarriage.

## Injuries to the Body of the Uterus

Apart from obstetrical rupture of the uterus, the only common gynaecological injury is perforation during dilatation and curettage, or during attempts to procure abortion.

Perforation is seldom dangerous unless the uterus is infected, or contains new growth, or unsterile instruments are used. In most cases it is only necessary to keep the patient under observation for a few days, and treatment is only needed if there is evidence of peritonitis.

## Stress Incontinence

Urinary incontinence on straining or coughing is termed stress incontinence, and is a common result of damage to the region of the bladder neck at delivery. Though often associated with prolapse, it is a separate injury.

The precise mechanism of bladder control in the female is uncertain. Radiological study shows that there is normally an angle between the posterior aspect of the urethra and the bladder base, and this angle is often lost in these cases. The angle is probably maintained by fibres of the levator ani which are inserted into the vagina and urethra, but the compressor urethrae muscle and striped muscle fibres in the wall of the urethra itself also assist in control. Whatever ,the normal mechanism, tightening of the structures below the urethro-vesical junction and elevation of the bladder base will often cure stress incontinence. Shortly after delivery, improvement may be gained by pelvic floor exercise and faradism, but cases that persist require operation. A diamond-shaped piece of the vaginal mucosa overlying the urethra is removed, to allow deep stitches to be placed so as to draw the paraurethral tissues together below the urethra; the vaginal skin is then sutured. Difficult cases require more extensive operations, such as that of Aldridge by which a sling formed from the aponeurosis of the external oblique muscle is drawn down behind the symphysis, to elevate and constrict the urethra. Alternatively, a strip of ox fascia or a free graft of fascia lata may be used for the sling.

Another method of elevating the bladder neck is by the Marshall-Marchetti operation, in which a small suprapubic incision is made and the anterior wall of the bladder is drawn up and fixed to the posterior aspect of the pubic bone.

## DISPLACEMENTS OF THE UTERUS
## AND VAGINA

### Prolapse

This term is applied to descent or protrusion of the vaginal walls or uterus.

**Aetiology.** Weakened pelvic supports (pp. 7, 8). Most cases (99 per cent) occur in parous women. (1) During pregnancy the pelvic supports are softened and hyperaemic. Return to normal may be delayed by sepsis, too frequent pregnancies, or inadequate rest after labour. Although early exercise assists muscle recovery injudicious strain will have the opposite effect. (2) During the labour the supports may be torn or overstretched, e.g. by prolonged straining or violent forceps delivery. (3) After the menopause the pelvic supports atrophy,

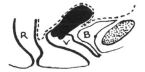

NORMAL

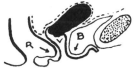

RECTOCELE _ CYSTOCELE

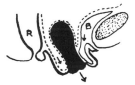

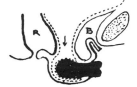

UTERINE DESCENT

Fig. 11. Types of prolapse.

and prolapse may first appear then; this is always the cause of the rare cases in nulliparae. (4) Poor general health will lower muscular tone. Prolapse is commoner in poorer women, though heavier work and larger families are also factors here.

B. Increased intra-abdominal pressure, or increased weight of the uterus may be contributory factors.

**Anatomy.** The lesions may be artificially subdivided:
A. Uterine descent (vault prolapse). This can only occur if

the cardinal ligaments are damaged. The vagina usually prolapses first, but in a few cases the uterus descends first and the vaginal walls follow. Once vaginal drag begins the supravaginal cervix becomes elongated by traction; while the vaginal cervix becomes oedematous, often with secondary infection or ulceration. Degrees of descent are: First, retroversion with descent of the cervix to the vaginal orifice. Second, cervix protruding. Third (or procidentia), uterus outside the vulva with complete vaginal inversion. In procidentia the prolapsed mass contains bladder, uterus and adnexae, peritoneal pouches which may contain gut, and drawn down rectal wall.

B. Anterior vaginal wall descent (Cystocele). This occurs with uterine descent, but can occur alone. The bladder fails to empty completely at micturition, and cystitis often occurs.

C. Posterior vaginal wall descent (Rectocele). If the perineal body is damaged the lower part of the posterior wall can prolapse, together with a pouch of the underlying rectal wall. The upper part of the posterior vaginal wall inevitably descends if the uterus descends.

D. Hernia of the recto-vaginal pouch (Enterocele). This often accompanies a rectocele, but may occur alone. This is a site at which prolapse may recur after operation.

**Symptoms.** There is a sensation of perineal weakness— 'bearing down'. Urinary symptoms include frequency, stress incontinence, and (only in cases of procidentia) retention. Discharge may occur from the exposed and oedematous cervix. Backache is occasionally relieved by treatment of prolapse, but is far more often found to be due to other causes.

**Treatment.** A. Palliative. Pessary treatment is never curative, and is inconvenient as the patient must have the pessary changed at intervals. It may be indicated for (1) patients unfit or too old for operation; (2) young women who hope for further pregnancy, but if symptoms are unrelieved by a pessary operation should not be withheld in such cases; (3) in early pregnancy.

Ring pessaries are used; those made of new plastic materials are better than rubber rings. The ring is compressed for insertion, and should be large enough to fill the vault, but should never cause discomfort. A ring is useless if the vaginal orifice is too relaxed to retain it, and often fails to control a cystocele. If a ring pessary will not serve, a cup and stem pessary can be used. Pessaries will not relieve stress incontinence.

B. Curative. Operative treatment is recommended whenever possible (see p. 122).

*Pregnancy after an operation for prolapse.* In most cases vaginal delivery with epistomy is best, but if stress incontinence has been successfully cured Caesarean section may be considered.

## Retroversion

In retroversion the uterine fundus is directed backwards. *Retroversion is a physical sign, not a disease.*

**Clinical Types.** A. 'Congenital retroversion.' As the uterus enlarges at puberty it may fall back instead of becoming anteverted. About 20 per cent of healthy women have retroversion of this type. Congenital retroversion does not cause backache or pelvic symptoms. If pregnancy occurs the retroverted uterus usually rises up uneventfully, but sometimes becomes incarcerated in the pelvis (see below). Congenital retroversion is sometimes associated with uterine hypoplasia, but if infertility or scanty periods occur they are not due to the retroversion but to the hypoplasia. Uncomplicated congenital retroversion practically never requires treatment, except for incarceration during pregnancy.

B. Puerperal retroversion. After delivery the uterus may become retroverted. This type of retroversion may be associated with menorrhagia and an abnormally bulky uterus (see p. 49). Backache may occur, but is more often due to poor posture and fatigue than to the retroversion. Dyspareunia occurs both because the ovaries lie in the recto-vaginal pouch, and also because the uterus itself is tender. When found at a postnatal examination retroversion may be corrected, and a pessary inserted until involution is complete; but if there are no symptoms or if the retroversion is known to have been present before pregnancy then no treatment is required.

C. Retroversion may be secondary to other pelvic lesions: (1) In prolapse. (2) Tumours such as fibromyomata may push the uterus backwards. (3) Fixed retroversion is due to adhesions from salpingitis, pelvic peritonitis or endometriosis. In all these cases there are symptoms, but these are *not* due to the retroversion, which is only incidental; and treatment is determined by the cause.

D. Retroversion and pregnancy. If pregnancy occurs in a retroverted uterus the uterus usually becomes anteverted as it enlarges into the abdomen. If the fundus fails to rise up the gravid uterus becomes incarcerated, and the cervix is directed sharply forwards, distorting the bladder base so that retention of urine occurs, usually at about 14 weeks. If unrelieved, retention with overflow, cystitis and miscarriage may occur. The care of these cases is an obstetrical problem, but may be briefly summarized: The bladder is slowly emptied with a catheter, and the uterus may then rise up spontaneously, but otherwise the fundus is pushed up (under anaesthesia if necessary) and a pessary inserted.

**Diagnosis.** In retroversion, the cervix is directed forwards, and the body of the uterus is felt through the posterior fornix and cannot be felt bimanually. The cervix of an acutely anteflexed uterus points forwards, but the fundus is directed forwards too.

The retroverted uterus must also be distinguished from other swellings felt through the posterior fornix such as uterine fibromyomata, ovarian tumours, pyosalpinx, pelvic abscess, pelvic haematocele, rectovaginal endometriosis, rectal carcinoma and faeces. Particular attention is paid to the history, whether the swelling is separate from the uterus, its consistency, and the direction of the cervix.

**Treatment.** Retroversion is corrected by pressing the fundus upwards with a finger in the posterior fornix, sometimes with the help of backwards pressure on the cervix. When corrected, the uterus is held forwards with a Hodge pessary. This is made of hard plastic material in varying sizes, and is roughly rectangular, but with one end curved to fit the posterior fornix, and slighter curves on the other sides.

Retroversion can also be treated by the operation of ventrosuspension, in which the round ligaments are used to hold the uterus forwards. Pregnancy can safely occur afterwards. Ventrofixation, in which the uterus is sewn to the anterior abdominal wall, should never be performed if there is any further possibility of pregnancy (see p. 127).

The indications for treatment may be summarized thus:

(1) Uncomplicated congenital cases: Treatment is not required.
(2) Puerperal cases (unless the retroversion was known to precede pregnancy): Pessary.
(3) Cases in parous women in whom the relation of retroversion to symptoms is doubtful: A pessary is tried; if symptoms are relieved operation may be considered.
(4) During pregnancy: If incarceration occurs, catheterization; replacement; occasionally a pessary is required.
(5) In cases secondary to other local disease: Correction at the time of operation for the disease.


## Acute Anteflexion

In some cases of uterine hypoplasia the uterus is sharply bent forwards, so that the fundus and cervix both point forwards (cochleate uterus). Scanty periods and infertility are due to the hypoplasia, not the antiflexion.


## Chronic Inversion of the Uterus

In inversion the uterus is turned inside out, and when it is complete the uterus lies in the vagina while the tubes and ovaries are dragged down into the cup formed by the inverted fundus. Acute puerperal inversion is a dangerous obstetrical accident. Such cases rarely persist as chronic puerperal inversion. Chronic inversion also occurs from traction on a fundal fibromyoma or sarcoma as the uterus contracts to expel the tumour.

Chronic inversion causes pain and bleeding, and on examination the fundus is absent from its normal situation and found in the vagina. The cervix often forms a tight constriction ring, so that replacement is difficult. Abdominal or vaginal operations to divide the constriction ring are possible, but the risk of sepsis makes vaginal hysterectomy a reasonable alternative. In cases due to a fibroid polyp, vaginal myomectomy is performed, taking care not to cut through the inverted fundus.

## Chapter 5

# INFLAMMATORY DISEASES

## VENEREAL DISEASES

### Gonorrhoea

**Transmission.** The cause is the diplococcus of Neisser, which is transmitted to adults by sexual intercourse. The newborn infant may be infected from the mother's genital tract, and in young children infection may also be transmitted by infected towels or hands. The gonococcus is a Gram-negative diplococcus, found within the pus cells of any discharge.

**Pathology.** Gonococci can penetrate the epithelium of urethra, cervix, or vestibular (Bartholin) glands; but do not infect the thick vaginal epithelium of the adult, though they may do so in children. From these primary sites infection spreads in the submucous tissues, causing acute inflammation with purulent discharge. Infection may spread upwards to uterus, tubes and peritoneum (see p. 50) and rarely spreads by the blood stream to joints, iris or endocardium.

**Symptoms and Signs.** The incubation period is from one to five days, usually two days. Purulent vaginal and urethral discharge appears, with frequency and pelvic discomfort. Severe pain or fever suggest spread to tubes or peritoneum. The initial symptoms may be slight or overlooked. Pus can be expressed from the urethra. Bartholin's glands may be swollen and tender, with the duct orifices evident as red puncta, and a Bartholin abscess may follow (p. 44). Discharge escapes from the inflamed cervical canal. Secondary vulvitis may occur. The vaginal epithelium is not involved in adults, but in children acute vaginitis may occur. The acute symptoms resolve spontaneously, but chronic cervicitis and salpingitis may persist, with arthritis and iridocyclitis as complications.

**Diagnosis.** In the acute stage swabs are taken from urethra and cervix after wiping away gross discharge, and smears and cultures prepared. Cultures are best put up immediately on warm serum agar, but swabs can be sent to the laboratory in

Stuart's transport medium. In the chronic stages secondary infection makes the discovery of the gonococcus in discharge more difficult, but the complement fixation test may then be positive.

**Treatment.** Care is taken in disposal of infected articles. All the antibiotics in common use are effective; an intramuscular injection of 2.4 g of procaine penicillin is commonly chosen, but some strains are found to be resistant and require other antibiotics. Local treatment is not required, but rest until acute symptoms have subsided reduces any risk of upward spread.

To confirm cure, swabs are taken just after the next three menstrual periods, with careful pelvic examination. A serological test for syphilis is done at the last examination.

## Syphilis

The following brief description only refers to the aspect of the disease encountered by the gynaecologist.

Syphilis is caused by the *treponema pallidum,* and almost invariably transmitted to the adult by sexual intercourse, though if an infected woman becomes pregnant her fetus may be infected.

The *primary chancre* is often unnoticed in women. It occurs most often on the labium or cervix, but may be anywhere on the lower genital tract, and occasionally on lip, nipple or finger. After an incubation period of 10-90 days (usually 28), an indurated papule appears, which breaks down to form an almost painless ulcer with firm margins, and persists for three to four weeks. There is often livid oedema around vulval chancres. The inguinal glands show painless, discrete, firm enlargement. Secondary infection may confuse these signs. The serological tests are not positive for 6-12 weeks after infection.

In the *secondary stage* malaise, anaemia, limb pains and slight fever may occur, with widespread enlargement of lymphatic glands. Eruptions appear on skin and mucous mambranes, with patchy alopecia and pigmentation. A common early rash consists of 'ham coloured' polymorphic macules, widespread over trunk and limbs, and without irritation; but many types of rash occur, including papules, pustules and scaly eruptions. White 'mucous patches' are seen on the buccal mucosa, and 'snail track' ulcers occur on the fauces. These are first covered by thick grey epithelium which separates to leave shallow ulcers. 'Condylomata lata' occur on the vulva and perineum as broad flat patches of epithelium that appear sodden and white.

In the *tertiary stage* the serious lesions of bones and joints, heart and blood vessels, nervous system and eyes occur. Gummata are rare in the pelvic organs.

**Diagnosis**. In the primary stage suspicious ulcers are examined for spirochaetes. The surface is cleaned with saline, and any serum that exudes is examined by dark ground method. The treponema may also be found in juice aspirated from a lymph gland. After 6-12 weeks the serological reactions such as the Kahn and Wassermann tests become positive, though treatment may alter the reactions.

**Treatment**. The primary sore and any discharge from secondary lesions are highly infectious. Sexual transmission becomes improbable after three years, but a woman can infect her child in utero for a longer period.

Most authorities now recommend treatment with penicillin alone, without using arsenic or bismuth. A typical course consists of 10 consecutive daily injections of 600,000 units of delayed action penicillin. Supervision is maintained for at least two years, and the patient should not marry until this period is past and serological and clinical examination negative.

### Soft Sore (Chancroid)

A venereal infection with *Haemophilus Ducreyii*, a small Gram-negative bacillus that is difficult to culture. The incubation period is 1-4 days. Multiple painful ulcers occur with undermined edges. The inguinal glands are swollen, matted, and often suppurate. The disease responds to several antibiotics, but probably best to streptomycin or chlortetra-cycline.

### Lymphogranuloma Venereum

A venereal infection with a filterable virus, for which the

Frei intradermal reaction is a specific test. The initial lesion is vesicular, but granulomatous masses appear later, with secondary ulceration, infection and fibrosis. The inguinal glands are matted together and may suppurate. Rectal stricture may follow from lymphatic spread. Chlortetracycline, streptomycin or chloramphenicol are effective for treatment, and aspiration of abscesses or excision of infected tissue is sometimes required.

### Granuloma Inguinale

A venereal disease usually only seen in the tropics. In the cells of the granulomatous masses capsulated bacteria can be found (Donovan bodies). Ulceration and scarring ultimately involve the whole vulval area. The disease responds to streptomycin, chlortetracycline or chloramphenicol.

Trichomoniasis, scabies, and infestation with pediculi may be venereally transmitted.

## INFLAMMATORY DISEASES OF THE VULVA

### Specific Infections

*Primary Chancre* (see p. 39).

In *gonorrhoea* urethritis and Bartholinitis occur, sometimes with vulval oedema.

*Chancroid (soft sore)* (see p. 40).

*Lymphogranuloma venereum and granuloma inguinale* (see above).

Streptococci or staphlococci cause *impetigo* or *furunculosis.*

Vulval *diphtheria* is rare. Membrane forms, antiserum is required.

*Monilial vulvitis* is due to infection with *Candida albicans.* It is common in diabetes, when there is glycosuria, and in pregnancy. The vulva is acutely inflamed and white patches occur, in which the mycelium can be found. It may be treated by local application of gentian violet (1 per cent solution) or with nystatin (antibiotic) pessaries and cream.

Vulval *tuberculosis* is very rare, and is almost invariably secondary to other pelvic tuberculous lesions.

*Herpes* virus causes a vesicular eruption which may be followed by ulceration. There is no specific treatment. Lesions may occur on the cervix. There may be an association between this infection and cervical cancer (see p. 63).

*Vulval warts* (condylomata acuminata) are caused by virus infection, but vaginal discharge seems to be a predisposing factor. They are usually multiple. Treat by coagulation with diathermy.

*Gangrenous vulvitis (noma pudendi)* is a rare but dangerous event in debilitated children, due to a mixed infection with streptococci and other organisms. Spreading gangrene occurs, with severe toxaemia. Suitable antibiotics are chosen according to the organisms found.

### Secondary Vulvitis

Occurs in cases of:
1. Vulval irritation from scratching (see pruritus, below).
2. Profuse vaginal discharge from any cause.
3. Urinary incontinence, especially with pyuria.
4. Diabetes, due to monilia which grows in the excreted sugar.

### Leukoplakia, Kraurosis and Chronic Vulvitis

Dermatologists are very critical of the use that gynaecologists have made of the terms leukoplakia and kraurosis in the past, but modern attempts to include all these conditions under a single heading are unhelpful. The following description tries to use dermatological terms correctly. For diagnosis biopsy and the help of the skin specialist may be necessary.

(1) Any persistent vaginal discharge will cause pruritus, and scratching may cause *lichenification* of skin. Adjacent parts of the perineum and thighs may be involved. Inflammatory changes cause thickening and oedema of the skin (not to be confused with true leukoplakia). The treatment is to cure the discharge, to give sedatives which are adequate to secure sleep, and local antipruritics to stop the scratching, such as zinc cream with 1 per cent phenol.

Anaesthetic creams (e.g. benzocaine) may be used, but there is some risk of sensitivity reactions. Hydrocortisone ointment (1 per cent) is often helpful.

(2) True *leukoplakia occurs in patches,* but is confined to the vulva. Many cases, but not all, occur in women who already have one of the other conditions listed here. There is severe pruritus. The involved skin is white and thickened. Epithelial proliferation occurs, with irregular downgrowth of papillae, and heaping up of swollen surface cells. Hyaline degeneration occurs in the dermis. *In many cases epithelioma follows,* and leukoplakic skin should be excised without delay.

(3) *Lichen sclerosus* is commonly mistaken for leukoplakia. Lesions may be found elsewhere on the body, and it may extend back to the anus. Soreness and pruritus occur. There are ivory coloured papules, with hyperkeratosis around hair follicles. The cause is unknown and treatment is symptomatic.

(4) *Kraurosis* (primary atrophy) is usually seen in post-menopausal women, whose complaint is of pain. The skin is atrophic, thin and dry, with a yellow or red colour. Shrinking of labia and contraction of the vaginal orifice ultimately occur. Some of these cases respond to oestrogens (stilboestrol 5 mg daily by mouth and oestrone ointment).

## Pruritus Vulvae

Vulval irritation is caused by:

(1) Urinary conditions: Glycosuria, pyuria, incontinence.
(2) Vaginal discharge from any cause.
(3) Rectal conditions: Haemorrhoids, thread worms.
(4) Pelvic congestion and leucorrhoea due to pregnancy or pelvic tumours.
(5) Skin diseases: Leukoplakia, lichen sclerosus, pediculi, scabies, allergic reactions, etc.
(6) Neurosis, usually as a sequel to some local cause.

Vulval irritation is maintained by scratching, and not infrequently by allergic response to applications used in treatment.

**Treatment**. Find the cause and remove it. In the meantime, sedatives, and local antipruritics are given to stop scratching, such as coal tar and lead lotion, 1 per cent gentian violet (for cases with sepsis), cinchocaine ointment (1 per cent), or 1 per cent phenol in zinc cream. Hydrocortisone ointment (1 per cent) may be used in cases due to sensitization. Excess soap and water should be avoided, oil being used for cleansing. In resistant cases, local injection of proctocaine in oil may give relief.

### Bartholinitis

*Acute Bartholinitis* may occur in gonorrhoea, but is far more often the result of infection by other organisms. There is local pain, and pus can be squeezed from the duct. A *Bartholin abscess* may follow, as a tender hot swelling under the posterior part of the labium minus. Systematic antibiotics and incision are required. Such abscesses tend to recur, and then the whole gland is excised, leaving the wound widely open to drain. A *Bartholin cyst* is due to blockage of the duct by secretion or previous inflammation, and the translucent cyst contains mucoid fluid. The treatment is by excision, or by opening the cyst and suturing its lining to the skin (marsupialization).

## VAGINITIS

Infection occurs more easily when the vaginal acidity is absent or lowered; before puberty or after the menopause, during menstruation or the puerperium.

### Infection with Trichomonas Vaginalis

This organism is a protozoon, about the size of a leucocyte, and actively motile by means of its flagella. It causes a profuse yellow purulent discharge, often containing minute bubbles. There may be small red erosions over the cervix and fornices, and severe secondary vulvitis. The infection is usually transmitted by intercourse, but sometimes by contaminated towels or water. The organism is detected by placing a little of the discharge in a drop of normal saline on a slide and searching for the motile organisms with a microscope.

**Treatment.** Nearly all cases respond to treatment with metronidazole ('Flagyl') 200 mg thrice daily by mouth for seven days. As recurrences are usually due to reinfection the sexual partner is given the same treatment. If this treatment fails stovarsol vaginal pessaries ('S.V.C.') may be used. One or more pessaries are inserted as high as possible at night and the treatment must be continued for at least six weeks to reduce the risk of recurrence. During this time intercourse is forbidden, because cross infection is common.

## Infection with Monilia (Candida) Albicans

This occurs most frequently during pregnancy, or with glycosuria, but may occur at other times. White patches are seen on the vagina or vulva, but in pregnancy the vagina may be filled with white semisolid masses of mycelium. The mycelial threads of the organisms are found by examining films of the discharge. Treatment is by insertion of nystatin pessaries (100,000 units). Painting with 1 per cent gentian violet is also effective treatment.

## Infection with Haemophilus Vaginalis

Some cases of vaginitis have been attributed to infection with this organism but it is doubtful whether it is a pathogen. It is a minute Gram-negative micro-aerophilic bacillus which is cultured with difficulty on media containing blood. It is easily killed by all the common antibiotics and antiseptics.

## Vulvo-Vaginitis of Children

In the absence of vaginal acidity infection with coliforms and various cocci may occur, especially if there is lack of hygiene, a foreign body, or infestation with thread worms. Monilial infection may occur, particularly if other bowel organisms have been killed by antibiotics. Trichomonads and gonococci may be transmitted indirectly by towels, clothing, etc.

Profuse yellow discharge with acute vulvitis occurs. The cause must be found, and appropriate antibiotics given for specific infections. Oestrogens will induce the development of a more resistant adult type of epithelium (e.g. stilboestrol 0.5 mg daily by mouth with a 1,000 unit oestrone pessary vaginally daily).

## Senile Vaginitis

This is a non-specific infection due to a variety of organisms that gain a foothold in the absence of the acid barrier, and may spread upwards to the endometrium (see p. 48). Vaginal stenosis may follow. There is thin purulent discharge, sometimes bloodstained. Treatment: 2 per cent lactic acid douches, with stilboestrol 1 mg daily by mouth, and 1,000 unit oestrone pessaries locally. The dose of stilboestrol is reduced as soon as possible, otherwise confusing uterine bleeding may occur.

## Vaginitis Secondary to Other Causes

May be due to:

(1) Any retained foreign body such as a pessary or tampon.
(2) Irritant douches or contraceptives.
(3) Urinary or rectal fistulae.
(4) Foul discharge from a neoplasm.

The treatment is to remove the cause, with antiseptic douches in the meantime.

## INFLAMMATORY DISEASES OF THE UTERUS

### Pathways of Infection

Normally there are no bacteria in the cervical canal or uterine cavity. Infection of the body of the uterus tends to die out after a few menstrual cycles, but often persists in the deep cervical glands. Causes of infection: (1) The great majority of cases follow abortion or labour, and are due to a variety of organisms, including streptococci, coliforms and staphylococci. The acute stages of these infections are an obstetric problem, and are not considered here. (2) Gonococci may ascend into the uterus, but infection only persists in the cervix. (3) Tubercle bacilli may infect both endometrium and muscle, by the blood stream. (4) Senile endometritis is due to ascending infection when the vaginal acidity falls. (5) Following gynaecological operations. (6) Infection of the prolapsed cervix. (7) Infection of necrotic neoplasms.

## Cervicitis and Cervical Erosion

**Acute Cervicitis**. May be puerperal or gonococcal.

**Chronic Cervicitis**. Follows acute cervicitis or may occur in the prolapsed uterus. The cervix is often patulous or lacerated, and may be fixed by paracervical fibrosis. The cervical mucosa is hypertrophic, sometimes forming polypi at the external os (see p. 62). Some of the cervical glands are distended with secretion and form 'Nabothian cysts' which may project on the vaginal surface. There is mucopurulent discharge which may cause an erosion (see below). Microscopical section shows fibrosis, with round cell and polymorphonuclear infiltration.

**Cervical Erosion** is secondary to cervical discharge and is not itself a primary inflammatory lesion, nor is it a true ulcer. An erosion is seen as a bright red velvety area extending from the external os over the vaginal surface of the cervix. If there is excessive alkaline cervical discharge, the pink stratified epithelium, whose normal environment is acid, is lost, and replaced by red columnar epithelium which grows out from the canal. The surface bleeds easily, but is not friable, and may be smooth or papillary.

Most erosions are not due to cervicitis, and some are seen in virgins ('congenital erosions'). In the fetus the columnar epithelium extends beyond the external os, but a more probable explanation of non-infective erosions is that there is an excessive discharge due to oestrogens. Erosions are common in women on 'the pill'. Erosions commonly occur during pregnancy and the puerperium and often resolve without treatment.

**Symptoms of Chronic Cervicitis**. Muco-purulent discharge occurs, and may cause vulvitis. The cervix is normally insensitive, but in chronic cervicitis may be tender on pressure, causing dyspareunia. Frequency is common.

**Treatment of Cervicitis and Erosion**. (1) The hot wire or diathermy cautery is used to lay open infected glands and coagulate the superficial epithelium of the cervical canal and over an erosion. This is best done with an anaesthetic, though it is possible without. Discharge increases for about seven days until sloughs separate and the superficial epithelium regenerates. Secondary haemorrhage occasionally occurs, but can be controlled by vaginal packing. Stenosis is an uncommon sequel of cauterization.

(2) Alternatively a porous 'pencil' soaked in concentrated zinc chloride solution can be inserted into the cervical canal (without anaesthesia) and left for two hours, so that the superficial tissues are coagulated and separate after a few days, when regeneration occurs from the deeper parts of the glands.

(3) Amputation of the cervix is unsatisfactory, as only part of the infected cervix is removed, and abortion may occur in a subsequent pregnancy.

(4) If there is associated uterine or tubal disease in parous women, total hysterectomy is recommended.

## Acute Endometritis and Metritis

May be puerperal, or a transitory event in gonorrhoea.

## Uterine Tuberculosis

Occurs in association with rubal infection. Tubercles are found in the endometrium, and there is often excessive or irregular menstrual loss. For diagnosis and treatment see p. 54.

## Senile Endometritis

May occur when the vaginal acidity falls after the menopause, by ascending infection with coliforms and streptococci. The uterus becomes lined with granulation tissue, and if the cervical canal is blocked becomes distended with pus (*pyometra*). Senile endometritis causes a thin bloodstained purulent discharge; but if pyometra supervenes, there may be no discharge but pelvic discomfort, and gradual enlargement of the uterus.

**Treatment.** The cervix is dilated, and a catheter introduced to allow drainage and the instillation of acriflavine in glycerine, while oestrogens are given as for senile vaginitis (p. 46). Pyometra will respond to the same treatment but often recurs, when hysterectomy is required.

(*Pyometra* may also be due to blockage of the cervix by carcinoma, or to stenosis after radium treatment, and these possibilities must always be considered.)

### Chronic Metritis and Subinvolution

In women over 40, especially parous women, it is common to find a symmetrical enlargement of the uterus, with menorrhagia, leucorrhoea and backache. The heavy uterus is often retroverted, and the wall is uniformly thick and rigid, with prominent vessels on the cut surface. The endometrium is often normal, but sometimes hypertrophic. This description may include more than one entity:

(1) Diffuse uterine hypertrophy occurs with cystic endometrial hyperplasia (p. 90). The clinical and pathological features of these cases are clearly defined.

(2) True (inflammatory) chronic metritis may persist as a rare sequel of acute metritis. Section shows fibrosis and round cell infiltration.

(3) Subinvolution. In any parous uterus section shows residual rings of elastic tissue around the blood vessels, which are remains of the elastica of the hypertrophied vessels of pregnancy. It is claimed that diffuse enlargement of the uterus is due to incomplete involution after pregnancy, and that the elastic deposits are greater in these cases.

(4) Diffuse adenomyosis (see p. 82).

The reason for the menorrhagia of the 'bulky uterus' is often obscure, as the endometrium may appear normal.

**Treatment.** An artificial menopause can be induced by placing 100 mg of radium in the uterus for 24 hours, with screenage equivalent to 1 mm of lead, but total hysterectomy is usually the best treatment, especially in parous women. Hormone treatment is not advisable or successful for these patients.

## SALPINGO-OÖPHORITIS

### Aetiology

(1) Infection of tubes and ovaries may follow delivery or abortion, when *streptococci* ascend from the placental site or a cervical laceration by the lymphatics or the cellular spaces. Puerperal infection by other organisms less commonly damages the tubes.
(2) *Gonococci* may ascend by the uterine lumen from a primary cervicitis.
(3) *Tuberculous* salpingitis may be due to blood spread from a distant focus, and may be either sequel or origin of tuberculous peritonitis.
(4) Any pelvic infection, such as appendicitis or an infected ovarian cyst, may secondarily involve the tube.

**Pathology.** Gonococcal salpingitis is usually acute in onset, streptococcal salpingitis may be acute or insidious, and tuberculous salpingitis is chronic.

In *acute salpingitis,* the tube is congested and oedematous. Pus escapes from the abdominal ostium, and in the streptococcal cases organisms also spread directly through the wall to cause pelvic peritonitis. Resolution may occur at this stage, but often swelling of the mucosa and adherence of its folds blocks the ends of the tube so that it becomes distended with pus, forming a thick-walled and retort-shaped *pyosalpinx.* Less active infection causes a *hydrosalpinx,* when the tube is equally distended, but with thin walls and clear fluid. The contents of a hydrosalpinx or long-standing pyosalpinx are usually sterile, but secondary infection with coliforms or other organisms may occur and cause an acute exacerbation. Salpingitis may also cause tubal blockage with thickened walls, but without distention (*interstitial salpingitis*).

The ovary is usually involved, and is often buried in adhesions and contains follicular cysts. Sometimes an infected tube comes to communicate with a small ovarian cyst to form a *tubo-ovarian cyst or abscess.* Salpingo-oöphoritis is nearly always bilateral, and the dense adhesions formed may hold the uterus in retroversion.

## Acute Gonococcal and Puerperal Salpingitis

**Symptoms and Signs.** In gonorrhoea upward spread to the tubes is often deferred until the succeeding menstrual period. Puerperal salpingitis is part of widespread pelvic inflammation, and often only recognized after some days of a febrile puerperium.

Severe symptoms arise when the peritoneum is involved. There is sharp lower abdominal pain, usually bilateral. The menstrual rhythm is often upset, and a profuse period occurs. There is a muco-purulent discharge from associated cervicitis, and often frequency. Much vomiting, or any prolonged change in bowel habit is unusual.

On examination there is fever (39°C+) and lower abdominal tenderness and resistance. There is extreme tenderness in both lateral vaginal fornices, which usually prevents precise examination, but inflammatory masses consisting of matted tubes and adjacent structures may be felt.

**Diagnosis.** Other acute abdominal conditions are considered, but especially (1) ectopic gestation (missed period, no fever, unilateral signs, pallor); (2) appendicitis (vomiting and constipation, furred tongue, right-sided signs, lower temperature); (3) torsion of an ovarian cyst (well-defined lump).

**Treatment.** Complete rest on a light diet with plenty of fluid. A full course of ampicillin is given, or other antibiotics that bacteriological investigation may suggest. Heat is applied to the abdomen, and after 48 hours, hot vaginal douches. Most cases respond to conservative treatment, and laparotomy is only required for cases in which the diagnosis is doubtful, or cases that fail to improve after some days (see below). Spreading peritonitis seldom occurs, so that conservative treatment is usually possible in the initial stage.

## Chronic Gonococcal and Puerperal Salpingitis

**Symptoms and Signs.** Chronic salpingitis may follow an

acute attack, or may have an insidious onset, especially after abortion or childbirth. Recurrent subacute attacks may occur, or there may be persisting pelvic pain and backache. Congestive premenstrual dysmenorrhoea occurs, and sometimes dyspareunia. There is often menorrhagia. Asociated cervicitis causes muco-purulent discharge. Persistent pain, sepsis and menorrhagia may cause general ill-health. Tubal blockage causes sterility. There may be no fever except in an exacerbation. There is usually cervicitis, and the uterus may be held in retroversion with fixed tender tubo-ovarian masses behind it, commonly bilateral, but of unequal size.

**Diagnosis.** Other causes of retroversion and other swellings in the recto-vaginal pouch are considered (see p. 35). Cases of ovarian endometriosis may be indistinguishable, with pain, sterility, menorrhagia and similar signs; but they have no cervicitis. Pelvic haematocele may also cause difficulty, but the history is different, and the uterus anteverted.

**Treatment.** A. Conservative. Comprises (1) treatment of anaemia and general health. (2) Pelvic heat, by diathermy or hot douches. (3) Antibiotics in exacerbations.

B. Laparotomy is recommended if there are recurrent acute attacks, if there are persistent symptoms that fail to respond to conservative treatment, or if there is a large pelvic mass. Infected tissue is excised, and as the cervix is often infected, total hysterectomy is often wise; it is sometimes possible to conserve some ovarian tissue. A pelvic abscess may be drained vaginally.

C. In a few cases salpingostomy or other plastic operations may subsequently be attempted for sterility due to blocked tubes, but success is infrequent.

## Tuberculous Salpingitis (see p. 54)

## Oöphoritis

Inflammation of the ovary follows and accompanies salpingitis and is due to the same causes. Other pelvic infections such as appendicitis may involve the ovary, and an ovarian cyst that becomes twisted or otherwise damaged may become infected. Oöphoritis sometimes occurs in mumps.

The ovary may contain single or multiple abscesses, or a tubo-ovarian abscess may occur (see above). In the chronic stages the ovary contains multiple follicular cysts, and is buried in dense adhesions which may cause sterility. Loculated collections of fluid in these adhesions may mimic ovarian cysts, both clinically and at operation. Excessive and frequent menstruation occurs.

The diagnosis and treatment are the same as for salpingitis.

## PELVIC PERITONITIS AND CELLULITIS

### Pelvic Peritonitis

Pelvic peritonitis may be caused by appendicitis, diverticulitis or infection of a carcinoma of the bowel. 'Gynaecological' types of infection are: (1) puerperal, most often due to streptococci or coliforms; (2) gonococcal; (3) pelvic tuberculosis; (4) infection of an ovarian cyst; (5) infection of a uterine growth; (6) infected haematoma, after operation or ectopic pregnancy.

In peritonitis an effusion occurs, which is usually localized by adhesions, and may then absorb, become encysted, or become an abscess. Subsequent adhesions may cause sterility and bind the uterus in retroversion.

The history varies with the cause, but the symptoms and signs of acute cases are fairly characteristic. There is severe lower abdominal pain, with vomiting and fever. Constipation is usual, but diarrhoea may occur if the bowel is irritated. The lower abdomen is tender and rigid, and there is tenderness and fullness in the vaginal fornices. If an abscess forms the temperature 'swings', the mass becomes more definite, then softens, and if left may point rectally or above the inguinal ligament.

Treatment varies with the cause. Most 'gynaecological' cases are localized and should be treated conservatively unless an abscess forms. Complete rest, chemotherapy, and heat to the abdomen are ordered. Hot douches or diathermy are unwise in the acute stage, and purges and enemas forbidden. If an abscess forms it can sometimes be drained through the posterior fornix.

## Pelvic Cellulitis (Parametritis)

In spite of text-book descriptions, pelvic cellulitis and peritonitis are not separate events but are usually combined in varying degree. Infection of pelvic cellular tissue nearly always follows abortion or delivery, and only rarely follows gynaecological operations or irradiation of infected neoplasms. Infection spreads by continuity in the cellular tissue.

The main features are pelvic discomfort, persistent fever and toxaemia, with the discovery of an indurated mass of 'woody' hardness in one or both lateral fornices. The induration fixes the cervix and may extend backwards in the utero-sacral tissue or upwards in the extraperitoneal tissues. Slow but complete resolution usually occurs, though an abscess may form, most frequently pointing above the inguinal ligament or into the rectum. Thrombophlebitis is a common complication. Sometimes fibrosis persists in the parametrium and fixes the cervix to one side.

**Treatment.** Complete rest, with full diet and attention to any anaemia. Hot douches or diathermy assist resolution, and antibiotics are used if the casual organism is susceptible. An abscess requires drainage.

## PELVIC TUBERCULOSIS

**Pathology.** Tubercle bacilli are thought to reach the female genital organs by the blood stream from a distant focus, although the primary focus is not always evident. The bacilli are usually of the human type. Infection of the pelvic organs occurs in tuberculous peritonitis, and conversely the pelvic organs may be the initial source of peritoneal infection. The tubes are the commonest site of the disease, and ovarian and uterine infections are fairly common, but infections of the cervix, vagina and vulva are very rare. In rare instances the lower tract is secondarily infected by descending infection.

Tuberculous pyosalpinx is retort-shaped and usually bilateral, contains caseous pus and has tubercles on the peritoneal surface. The abdominal ostium is blocked by the adherence of fimbriae, but these are not indrawn, as they are in gonococcal cases. Ovarian abscesses occur. In the uterus tubercles are found in both muscle and endometrium, often with little gross change. In the cervix, vagina and vulva undermined ulcers occur.

**Symptoms and Signs**. Pelvic tuberculosis is commonest in young adults. The onset is insidious with malaise and slight fever. There may be pelvic pain and congestive dysmenorrhoea, and sometimes more acute attacks due to secondary infection with other organisms. Leucorrhoea and menorrhagia are common, though amenorrhoea occurs in advanced cases. The signs are those of chronic salpingitis (p. 51) though without history of previous gonococcal or puerperal infection.

Ascites sometimes occurs, when the first complaint may be of abdominal swelling. Tapping yields a sterile bloodstained fluid, and diagnosis from malignant ovarian disease may be difficult. In the plastic form of tuberculous peritonitis, the abdomen has a 'doughy' feel.

Many cases of tuberculous endometritis are only discovered at endometrial biopsy during investigation of sterility or menorrhagia, and biopsy may be required to diagnose the rare ulcers of the lower genital tract.

In about one-fifth of the cases X-ray of the chest shows active disease. In the female coincident infection of the urinary track is not common. Advanced cases become cachectic, with fever, diarrhoea, and vomiting.

**Treatment**. For patients with active pulmonary infection of widespread abdominal disease sanatorium treatment is ordered with a full course of chemotherapy, usually consisting of a three months' course of streptomycin injections (1 g daily) combined with sodium para-aminosalicylate (12 g daily in cachets) and isoniazid (200 mg daily). PAS and isoniazid are continued for about two years.

Surgical treatment is only advised for cases with symptoms or localized masses which do not respond to chemotherapy, when hysterectomy and bilateral salpingo-oöphorectomy is usually required. Sometimes the diagnosis is only made on opening the abdomen for ascites or chronic sapingitis, and then diseased organs are removed if this can easily be done; but it is most dangerous to attempt to free widespread plastic adhesions to bowel.

## Chapter 6

# TUMOURS

## TUMOURS OF THE VULVA, URETHRA AND VAGINA

### Vulval Tumours

**Benign Neoplasms.** *Fibromata* and *Lipomata* are often pedunculated and are easily excised. *Papillomata* (vulval warts), are usually inflammatory rather than neoplastic, and are caused by virus infection, although vaginal discharge appears to be a predisposing factor. Such condylomata often clear up when the discharge is treated, but can otherwise be excised with diathermy. *Hidradenoma* is a rare benign solid tumour that arises from sweat glands. *Pigmented moles* occasionally give rise to *melanomata*; if there is any suspicion they should be widely excised; minor inadequate surgery is dangerous. *Endometriomata* may occur (p.81). *Varicosities of vulval veins* (vulval varices) are not neoplasms, but are mentioned here for convenience. They first appear during pregnancy, but may afterwards persist, and can be treated by injection with sodium morrhuate, or by excision.

**Epithelioma of the Vulva.** *Pathology.* Vulval carcinoma occurs most frequently in elderly women and often follows leukoplakia. It is a squamous-celled growth, with the rare exception of adenocarcinoma arising in Bartholin's gland. The growth most frequently starts on the labium majus, but also occurs on the clitoris, labia minora or near the urethra. When first seen the growth is usually ulcerated, but papillary and nodular types occur, and growth may also begin in a deep leukoplakic fissure. The inguinal lymphatic glands are soon involved, with subsequent spread to the iliac glands.

*Symptoms.* There is often long-standing pruritus from leukoplakia. A nodule appears which breaks down to form an ulcer with everted edges, and there is bloodstained discharge. Pain is due to secondary sepsis, or to involvement of deep structures. The inguinal glands are enlarged by metastases or sepsis. Diagnosis is from other causes of vulval ulceration (p. 41).

*Treatment.* In operable cases the whole vulva is excised with bilateral dissection of the inguinal, femoral and iliac glands (p. 122). Radical surgery gives much better results than radiotherapy, although this may be used for recurrences.

**Malignant Melanoma** is rare. When possible, the vulva and pigmented tumour is excised with the lymphatic glands, but the prognosis is very bad.

### Urethral Tumours

**Urethral Caruncle.** A caruncle appears at the posterior lip of the urethral orifice as a small red pedunculated swelling, sometimes very tender. There may be pain on micturition and dyspareunia, with slight bleeding.

Caruncles consist of granulation tissue, or of what appears to be vascular adenomatous tissue. Both types are due to tissue proliferation in response to local infection, though a few caruncles may be true adenomata of glands in the urethral floor.

*Treatment.* Excision. Any local or urinary infection must be dealt with. Caruncles often recur.

**Prolapse of the Urethral Mucosa.** To be distinguished from a caruncle. The swelling involves the whole circumference of the orifice. If causing symptoms, the redundant mucosa is excised.

**Carcinoma of the Urethra.** Very rare, and there is little fear of a caruncle becoming malignant. Both squamous-celled carcinoma and adenocarcinoma occur. If low down the treatment is as for vulval carcinoma; if high up radical urethrocystectomy is required.

### Vaginal Tumours

**Primary Carcinoma.** A rare tumour of the elderly, that resembles carcinoma of the cervix, with ulceration and bleeding. Treated with radium. Carcinoma *in situ* may occur in association with a similar lesion on the cervix (p. 63).

**Secondary Carcinoma** may follow uterine carcinoma. There may be direct spread from the cervix, or metastasis from carcinoma of the body of the uterus, sometimes as an isolated suburethral nodule. Vaginal recurrence after hysterectomy for cancer may occur, and is treated with radium.

**Secondary Chorion-epithelioma** occurs as a purple vascular tumour (p. 70).

**Endometrioma of the Recto-Vaginal Septum** (see p. 82).

**Gaertner's Cyst** (see p. 22).

## TUMOURS OF THE UTERUS

### Benign Tumours

**Fibromyomata.** *Pathology.* Fibromyomata are the commonest of all uterine tumours. They are usually found after the age of 30, and never develop for the first time after the menopause. They are more common in nulliparae.

Fibroids occur 15 times more often in the body of the uterus than in the cervix. Seedlings first appear in the uterine wall, and grow slowly, compressing the surrounding tissue to form a capsule. The tumours are gradually extruded from their initial *interstitial* position, towards the uterine cavity (to become *subendometrial*), or towards the peritoneal surface (to become *subperitoneal*); and in either case may become pedunculated. Fibromyomata are often multiple, and may grow to enormous size.

Fibroids are benign. Small tumours consist of smooth muscle fibres (myomata) but large tumours also contain fibrous tissue (fibromyomata). They are whiter in colour than the surrounding muscle, and their whorled structure can be seen with the naked eye. The tumours tend to outgrow their blood supply and then to show degenerative changes, although enormous hypertrophy of the uterine vessels occurs.

Fibromyomata may distort or displace the uterus, pushing it forwards or into retroversion, or to one side.

(a) Subendometrial fibroids first project into the uterine cavity so that the endometrial area is enlarged; and may then become pedunculated, when the uterus contracts to expel the polyp through the dilated cervix. Chronic uterine inversion may follow.

(b) Interstitial fibroids also distort the uterine cavity and increase the endometrial area. A fibroid in the cervical wall may greatly elongate the cervical canal and displace the body of the uterus upwards.

(c) Subperitoneal fibroids are often pedunculated.

(d) Cervical fibroids grow between the layers of the broad ligament displacing the uterus upwards or laterally and sometimes displacing or compressing the ureter.

In many cases not only is the uterine cavity enlarged, but the endometrium is hypertropic, and the uterine muscle may show diffuse hyperplasia. The ovaries often contain follicular cysts.

*Aetiology.* The aetiology of fibromyomata is obscure. On the inconstant evidence of the changes in the ovaries and the endometrium it is suggested that fibroids represent an abnormal response to oestrogens, although it is not possible to explain why the reaction is localized to certain parts of the muscle. The associated sterility, which is far from absolute, may be due to ovarian or endometrial abnormalities. Fibroids are very common in negresses.

## Secondary changes

(1) Degenerative changes are common as fibroids tend to overgrow their blood supply. *Atrophy,* which is seldom more then partial, occurs after a natural or artificial menopause, and sometimes after pregnancy. *Hyaline degeneration* is common in large or pedunculated tumours, and is without clinical significance. The connective tissue is first involved, with subsequent atrophy of muscle fibres. Cystic degeneration may follow. *Fatty degeneration* first involves the muscle fibres, and proceeds to *calcareous degeneration,* when the fat breaks down to soaps that take up calcium salts. This change is most common after the menopause. X-ray examination will

show calcification. *Red degeneration* is due to a relatively acute interference with blood supply, and is usually but not invariably seen during pregnancy. Possibly the rapid growth of the uterus kinks the capsular vessels: at any rate these vessels are often thrombosed. The tumour swells, softens, and becomes pinkish-red in colour. On microscopical examinarion a few surviving fibres are seen lying among dead fibres. Acute symptoms of fever, pain and vomiting occur. *Cystic degeneration* follows hyaline or red degeneration, and irregular cavities containing serous fluid appear.

(2) *Torsion* of a pedunculated fibroid, or of a whole tumour mass with the uterus may occur, causing acute pain, shock and vomiting. The tumour may become necrotic from loss of blood supply, or the tumour may acquire a 'parasitic' blood supply from omental adhesions

(3) *Infection* of a fibroid may occur after torsion; or the capsule of a submucous fibroid may be damaged, when infection can occur and the necrotic tumour is slowly extruded.

(4) *Impaction.* A tumour that fills the pelvis and displaces the bladder (especially a cervical fibroid) may cause urinary retention. Bowel symptoms are surprisingly rare. Impaction often occurs at a menstrual period or during pregnancy, but may also occur after the menopause when an abdominal tumour shrinks and suddenly sinks into the pelvis.

(5) *Malignant change.* Less than 0.2 per cent of fibroids become sarcomatous. The change is most common in large tumours. There is rapid enlargement, with pain, ascites and sometimes irregular or postmenopausal bleeding.

(6) *Fibromyomata and pregnancy.* Fibroids may cause sterility or abortion; or obstructed labour if situated in the lower uterine segment. Red degeneration, torsion and impaction are more frequent in pregnancy, and a fibroid is sometimes damaged and infected during labour.

*Symptoms. Many fibroids do not cause symptoms and do not require treatment.* The commonest symptom is *menorrhagia,* caused by endometrial hyperplasia or enlargement of the endometrial surface, or interference with uterine contractions. Menstrual loss is increased and prolonged, and the cycle is eventually shortened; severe anaemia may result. Postmenopausal bleeding does not occur unless the tumour is extruded as a polyp, or becomes sarcomatous. *Leucorrhoea* may occur. *Pain* is unusual with uncomplicated fibroids, but congestive dysmenorrhoea may occur, or uterine colic during the expulsion of a polyp. Pain occurs with the following complications: red degeneration, torsion, infection, sarcomatous change. With impaction painful *retention* occurs. (Pain associated with fibroids is often due to coincidental endometriosis.) The discovery of a large *abdominal tumour* is sometimes the only complaint.

*Signs.* Large tumours are felt on abdominal examination as hard painless tumours which rise up out of the pelvis. The tumour may be single and rounded, or consist of a group of rounded bosses. It is dull to percussion and no free fluid is evident. On auscultation a uterine souffle may be heard, as a result of the rich flow through the uterine vessels. On pelvic examination, the cervix is found to move laterally with the tumour mass.

Smaller tumours are found on pelvic examination as hard painless tumours attached to the uterus, though a pedunculated soft fibroid may simulate an ovarian tumour. A solitary interstitial fibroid is difficult to recognize as the uterine outline is smooth, although enlarged.

*Diagnosis.* An interstitial fibroid with degenerative softening may be difficult to distinguish from the pregnant uterus, but there is no amenorrhoea, nor is there cervical softening. In difficult cases pregnancy tests may be required.

Ovarian tumours are usually cystic, but a solid tumour may be mistaken for a pedunculated fibroid.

In cases of fibroids with postmenopausal bleeding the possibility of uterine cancer (especially of the body of the uterus) must be considered, and this is far commoner than sarcomatous change in fibroids.

Inflammatory masses and endometriosis may cause bleeding, but are tender, and less well defined than fibroids.

*Treatment.* Small symptomless fibroids do not require treatment, but large tumours nearly always need to be removed. Treatment is urgently required for torsion or impaction, is essential for menorrhagia or suspected sarcoma, and is sometimes required for pain or sterility. The symptoms of red degeneration usually resolve with rest, though the pain may be severe enough to need morphia for relief.

Most cases are treated *surgically*. (1) Polypoid tumours are excised by vaginal myomectomy. (2) Abdominal myomectomy is performed whenever possible in nulliparae under 40, or in parous women who desire further children. The operation is more difficult than hysterectomy and fibroids may afterwards recur (p. 127). (3) Abdominal hysterectomy is performed in the majority of cases (p. 126).

**Endometrioma.** (See p. 82).

**Endometrial Polypi.** *Pathology.* These are single adenomata, though histologically indistinguishable from the multiple polypi that occur in cases of cystic endometrial hyperplasia (p. 90). They are most common near the menopause, but occur in both younger and older women. Usually they arise near the internal tubal orifice, as soft pink tumours less than 1 cm in diameter, often flattened, and sometimes with a stalk that is long enough to allow them to reach the cervix. On section they are found to have a covering of endometrium, though squamous metaplasia often occurs. The polyp has an oedematous stroma, containing endometrial glands, some of which are cystic, and often showing incomplete response to the ovarian hormones. Secondary infection is common. Malignant change is rare, but occasionally occurs.

*Diagnosis.* Menorrhagia, leucorrhoea and sometimes irregular bleeding occur. Uterine colic or detectable enlargement are not seen. Diagnosis is only possible after dilating the cervix.

*Treatment.* The polypi are curetted away.

**Cervical (Mucous) Polypi.** *Pathology.* These occur at all ages, and may occur during pregnancy. Some of them are not true neoplasms, but are the result of proliferation of the endocervical epithelium in response to infection or oestrogens. Small soft pink polypi appear at the external os. On section they are found to consist of oedematous stroma containing glands resembling those of the cervix, and covered by tall columnar endocervical epithelium. Squamous metaplasia and secondary infection are common.

*Diagnosis.* There is discharge due to chronic cervicitis, and slight irregular bleeding from the polyp, which may be so soft that it is difficult to palpate, but is easily seen with a speculum.

*Treatment.* Polypi are easily removed, but the cervicitis must also be treated (p. 47).

**Placental (Fibrinous) Polypi.** These are not neoplastic, but occur when a fragment of chorionic tissue is retained after abortion or delivery, and layers of blood clot are deposited on the retained tissue. The mass becomes pedunculated as the uterus contracts to expel it. Irregular bleeding occurs. The polyp is removed with ovum forceps.

*Note.* The following uterine polypi occur:
A. Cervical: (1) Mucous (adenomatous). (2) Fibromyomatous. (3) Carcinomatous. (4) Sarcomatous. (5) Nabothian (see p. 47).
B. Corporeal: (1) Endometrial (adenomatous). (2) Fibromyomatous. (3) Placental. (4) Carcinomatous. (5) Sarcomatous.

## Malignant Tumours

**Carcinoma of the cervix.** *Aetiological Factors.* The commonest age for the growth to appear is between 40 and 50, but many cases are seen in older and younger women. About 95 per cent of the patients are parous. The incidence is increased in women of low socio-economic status and in some parts of Africa, Asia and S. America. The incidence in Europe appears to be falling. There is much to suggest that the causative factor is transmitted by coitus. The disease is almost unknown in virgins. It is more common with early marriage or coitus, and in women with many sexual partners. It is rare in Jews; although it has been suggested that this is because of male circumcision, careful studies of this and other races suggest that better sexual hygiene is a more likely explanation. The virus of herpes genitalis is associated with the tumour, but is not necessarily the cause of it.

A pre-invasive stage (carcinoma *in situ*) of several years' duration procedes the development of many cases of invasive cancer. Pre-invasive cancer does not cause symptoms and can only be discovered by careful examination of vaginal smears and biopsies. It is not yet known whether all, or only some of the cases, eventually progress to become invasive.

*Pathology.* The growth usually arises from the squamous epithelium of the portio vaginalis, but sometimes arises from the columnar epithelium of the cervical canal or glands. The growth first appears as a nodule, the cells of which infiltrate into the cervix, and also project from the surface, and either of these processes may predominate. As the growth soon outgrows its blood supply, necrosis and secondary infection follow, with bleeding and foul discharge. The friable growth breaks away to leave an ulcer crater, which progressively extends. Endocervical carcinoma grows in the canal and first expands the cervix, but subsequent spread is in the same manner. Cervical carcinoma spreads by:

A. *Local Spread.* The growth invades the adjacent vaginal vault. Lateral spread into the broad ligament fixes the cervix, and in later stages may obstruct the ureter. Anterior spread reaches the bladder, and in late stages necrosis causes a vesicovaginal fistula. Posterior spread first involves the uterosacral ligaments, and later the rectum, and may cause a rectovaginal fistula. Upward spread is often limited, but obstruction to the cervical canal may cause a pyometra.

B. *Lymphatic spread* may be early or late. The growth spreads to the iliac glands on the pelvic side wall and obturator fossa, and also backwards to the sacral glands.

C. *Blood spread* causes distant metastases, but is not common until late in the disease.

D. *Vaginal implantation* perhaps occurs, though lymphatic spread may equally explain the isolated vaginal metastases that are sometimes seen.

*Histology:* Ninety-five per cent of cervical carcinomata arise from squamous cells. This would be expected in growths that arise from the superficial squamous epithelium; but is also true for growths that start in the canal, probably because the columnar epithelium first undergoes metaplasia. The cells are often undifferentiated so that intercellular 'prickles' are not often seen; and cell nests are unusual as keratinization does not occur. The most active growths consist of spindle-shaped cells with little resemblance to normal epithelial cells. The remaining five per cent of growths are adenocarcinomata.

*Vaginal Cytology.* Early cancer does not cause symptoms, but at this stage exfoliated cancer cells may be recognized in secretion aspirated from the posterior fornix or in a smear prepared after scraping the cervix with a spatula. Routine examination of women aged 30 or more yields about 3 per 1,000 positive smears (invasive or pre-invasive). The discovery of suspicious cells merely indicates the urgent need for biopsy by excising the whole squamo-columnar junction with a subjacent cone of tissue, including most of the cervical canal.

*Symptoms.* Once ulceration has occurred there is *slight irregular bleeding, especially on examination* or intercourse; and diagnosis should be made at this stage, or even earlier by vaginal cytology. Unfortunately cases are often seen when necrosis and infection have caused bloodstained purulent foul discharge, or sometimes profuse bleeding.

Pain is a late symptom, due to spread of infection, to pyometra, or to extensive spread of growth. With bladder involvement there is frequency, and sometimes haematuria, and finally incontinence if a fistula forms. Uraemia from ureteric obstruction or ascending infection may be the final cause of death. Anaemia and cachexia occur in advanced cases.

*Signs.* In a really early case biopsy is necessary for diagnosis, but many cases are seen when the diagnosis is dreadfully obvious on clinical examination. The commonest discovery is a *crater* replacing part or whole of the cervix, with friable tissue in the base and edges. The growth is softer than the normal cervix, a probe will sink into it, and it bleeds on touching. With a speculum, infected necrotic tissue is seen.

Sometimes a *hypertrophic mass* of growth ('cauliflower type') is found, but the tissue is equally friable.

There may be no external evidence of *endocervical* carcinoma, but the cervix is distended to a barrel shape, and friable growth is revealed if the cervix is dilated.

In very early cases a small nodular area or ulcer is seen. Suspicious areas do not stain brown when painted with Lugol's iodine solution, in contrast to normal mucosa (Schiller's test).

*Stages of Cervical Carcinoma.* An international clinical

classification is in use. In brief: Stage 0, pre-invasive carcinoma. Stage I, confined to the cervix. Stage IIa, spread to vaginal vault. Stage IIb, spread to parametrium, but cervix not fixed. Stage III, spread to lower two-thirds of vagina, or parametrial spread with cervix fixed. Stage IV, metastases outside pelvis, or involvement of bladder or rectum.

*Late Diagnosis.* An ulcerated growth is to be distinguished from an erosion or an ulcer due to a retained pessary. Both erosion and cancer bleed on touch, but the base of an erosion is firm, not friable. If there is the slightest doubt biopsy is essential.

A polypoid growth is to be distinguished from other polypi, which are not friable. Section is essential.

*Prognosis.* With treatment, the five-year survival rate for Stage I growths is about 75 per cent, for Stage II growths about 50 per cent, and for Stage III and IV growths (together) about 10 per cent.

*Treatment of Pre-invasive Carcinoma.* If the tumour has been completely removed by biopsy the case may be followed up by repeated smears. Otherwise the safest course is to remove the uterus with a wide vaginal cuff. The ovaries can be left. This treatment can occasionally be deferred for a time until a pregnancy is achieved or completed.

*Treatment of Invasive Carcinoma.* The choice between radiotherapy and surgical treatment for operable cases is as hotly debated today as ever. The introduction of new and more powerful sources of radiation has been paralleled by a revival of interest in surgical techniques. Approximately equal results are obtained by the best exponents of the two methods, and the aim must be to select the best treatment for the individual case, perhaps by combined attack.

Many gynaecologists believe that radium offers better results than surgery, even for early cases. The immediate risk (due to septic complications) is very small, and the method can be used for all but the most advanced cases, in which there is a risk of precipitating fistula formation. Radium does not effectively irradiate glands on the pelvic wall, and deep X-ray therapy is therefore directed at these fields.

On the other hand, because a few cases with small primary

growths are found to have involved glands, and as there is some doubt whether X-ray treatment will sterilize these glands, some surgeons advise Wertheim's operation for the early cases.

*Stockholm Method of Radium Application.* Three applications are made, with a week between the first and second, and a fortnight between the second and third. At each application 40 mg of radium element are placed in the uterus, in a tubular container with screenage equivalent to 3 mm of lead. Seventy milligrammes of radium are distributed in the vaginal vault, in suitably shaped containers, with the same screenage. Gauze packing is used to hold the containers in place. Each application is left in place 22 hours, and an indwelling catheter is required until the pack is removed. The *Manchester method* is similar in principle, though the containers are devised so as to make dose calculations easier.

*Wertheim's Hysterectomy* is a difficult procedure only suitable for fit patients with operable growths (Stages I and II). It differs from an ordinary total hysterectomy in the following particulars. The ureter is fully exposed and retracted laterally so that the cardinal ligaments can be divided far out. The uterus, tubes and ovaries, broad ligaments, and upper third of the vagina are removed with as much of the adjacent cellular tissue as possible. Iliac and obturator lymphatic nodes are dissected out. Especial dangers are shock, bleeding from deep veins, and injury to the ureters or bladder.

*Schauta's operation* is an extended vaginal hysterectomy. The lymphatic glands cannot be removed, and for that reason it has few exponents in Britain.

In advanced cases only palliative treatment is possible, with drugs to relieve pain, although even more extensive operations (*pelvic exenteration*) in which the rectum or bladder is removed with the uterus are occasionally possible. In cases with severe pain intrathecal injection of alcohol to block sensory pathways may be considered.

**Carcinoma of the Body of the Uterus.** *Aetiological factors.* Usually but not invariably seen after the menopause. About half of the patients are nulliparous. There is some association with obesity and diabetes. It is suggested that some cases may be due to oestrogenic action because endometrial cancer may occur with granulosa cell tumours (see p. 74). and may sometimes follow endometrial hyperplasia. Endometrial cancer is often associated with fibromyomata, but probably only because both conditions are common in nulliparae.

*Pathology.* The growth arises from the endometrium, and in 95 per cent of cases is a columnar-celled carcinoma, often a well-differentiated adenocarcinoma, though undifferentiated types occur. The remaining five per cent of cases are squamous celled carcinomata.

The growth is usually found as a polypoid mass in the upper uterine cavity which eventually becomes necrotic, though infection is late as the situation is protected. In other cases there is less outgrowth, and ulceration predominates. The growth spreads by:

A. *Local spread.* The muscle wall is infiltrated, and ultimately penetrated; though the thick wall confines the growth for a time. Downward spread is limited, but the internal os may be blocked by growth, when pyometra follows.

B. *Lymphatic spread* chiefly follows the ovarian lymphatics to reach the glands around the aorta. In advanced cases the lymphatics around the uterine vessels are also involved, and exceptional spread occurs in lymphatics that accompany the round ligament to reach the inguinal glands. Ovarian metastases are common, by lymphatic pathways.

C. *Blood spread* is not prominent, but widespread metastasis may occur in late stages.

D. *Vaginal implantation* may occur, sometimes low down near the urethra.

*Symptoms.* The first symptom is bloodstained discharge, usually though not invariably occurring after the menopause. Profuse bleeding is less common than with cervical cancer. When infection of the growth occurs the discharge becomes purulent and foul. Slight pain may be due to uterine distention by growth or pyometra, but severe pain is a late event that only occurs when there is extensive spread. Finally, cachexia occurs.

*Signs.* The uterus often shows little clinical enlargement;

but in a minority of cases it is grossly enlarged by a large florid growth, by a pyometra, or more commonly because the growth arises in a fibromyomatous uterus.

*Diagnosis* depends on diagnostic curetting. Cancer cells may be found in a vaginal smear, but this test does not replace biopsy. Senile endometritis, endometrial polyp, or fibromyomatous polyp can only be distinguished after dilatation of the cervix. A granulosa cell tumour of the ovary will cause postmenopausal bleeding, but the ovarian tumour may be palpable, and the endometrium shows oestrogenic and not neoplastic change. Confusion may also arise in cases which have been given oestrogens.

*Prognosis.* With treatment the five-year survival rate is over 60 per cent.

*Treatment.* Ordinary total hysterectomy with bilateral salpingo-oöphorectomy and removal of a wide cuff of vagina gives fairly good results, but a few surgeons advocate Wertheim's hysterectomy, as lymphatic glands are sometimes involved. Radium is often inserted before operation to reduce the risk of recurrence in the vaginal vault.

This growth is radiosensitive, and in patients who are unfit for operation radium can be used as an alternative, though the results of surgical treatment are better.

Progestogens in large doses (e.g. $17\alpha$-hydroxyprogesterone caproate 5 g weekly intramuscularly) will cause remission of the growth in some cases.

**Sarcoma of the Uterus.** *Pathology.* Uterine sarcoma is an uncommon tumour. Sarcomatous change occurs in 0.2 per cent of fibromyomata, especially in large tumours near the time of the menopause, and although rare this is yet the commonest type of sarcoma. It is usually a spindle-shaped sarcoma. The histological evidence of malignancy may be doubtful even when the clinical course is certain.

Sarcoma of the endometrium is often a soft large vascular tumour that distends the uterine cavity and consists of round cells.

*Clinical Features.* Irregular and free uterine bleeding. The tumour grows rapidly, with pain, ascites and cachexia. Diagnosis usually depends on the microscopical section.

*Treatment.* Uterus and adnexae are removed, and X-ray therapy is given. The prognosis is bad.

**Mesodermal Mixed Tumours.** Although uncommon, these tumours are less rare than was formerly believed. They arise from the primitive mesoderm from which the Müllerian tract is developed. They are chiefly sarcomatous, but may contain mixed elements, including striped muscle, cartilage or carcinomatous tissue.

In adults the tumour grows as a large fleshy mass in the uterine cavity. A rare variety is the botryoid (grape-like) sarcoma of the cervix, usually seen in children. The tumours cause bleeding. They must be removed as radically as possible, but even with additional radiotherapy the prognosis is very bad.

**Chorion-epithelioma.** *Pathology.* This highly malignant tumour follows hydatidiform mole, or rarely a normal pregnancy. It is an extremely vascular tumour containing cells resembling those of chorionic trophoblast. The ovaries may contain non-malignant theca lutein cysts (see p. 72). Widespread metastases occur, especially in lungs and vagina.

*Diagnosis.* After delivery or removal of a hydatidiform mole a quantitative test for chorionic gonadotrophin is performed at two-monthly intervals for two years. If the test fails to become negative, or becomes positive again, or if there is uterine bleeding, then chorionepithelioma should be suspected. Curettage may reveal growth, and the lungs should be X-rayed for metastases. Vaginal recurrences occur as vascular purple nodules.

*Treatment.* If the uterus and ovaries are not fixed by extension of the growth they are removed. Patients with more extensive disease, distant metastases or recurrences are treated with folic acid antagonists (Methotrexate 0.5 mg/kg daily for five days). Courses, often combined with mercaptopurine, are repeated unless there are severe toxic symptoms or agranulocytosis occurs.


## TUMOURS OF THE OVARY

Without knowledge of aetiology, in ignorance of the tissue

from which many ovarian tumours arise, and with small distinction between benign and malignant varieties of some tumours, classification of ovarian tumours is unsatisfactory. The following table is simple and practical:

A. Distension cysts of the follicular apparatus.
    (1) Follicular cysts.    (2) Lutein cysts.

B. Cystic and solid neoplasms:

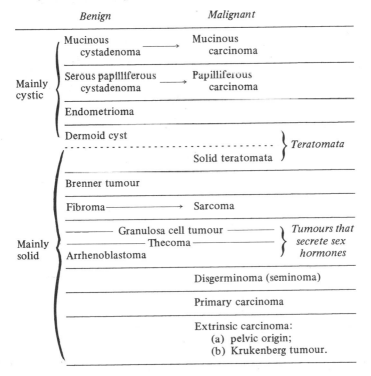

|  | *Benign* | *Malignant* |
|---|---|---|
| Mainly cystic | Mucinous cystadenoma → | Mucinous carcinoma |
|  | Serous papilliferous cystadenoma → | Papilliferous carcinoma |
|  | Endometrioma |  |
|  | Dermoid cyst | } *Teratomata* |
|  |  | Solid teratomata |
| Mainly solid | Brenner tumour |  |
|  | Fibroma → | Sarcoma |
|  | —— Granulosa cell tumour —— | } *Tumours that secrete sex hormones* |
|  | —— Thecoma —— |  |
|  | Arrhenoblastoma |  |
|  | Disgerminoma (seminoma) |  |
|  | Primary carcinoma |  |
|  | Extrinsic carcinoma: (a) pelvic origin; (b) Krukenberg tumour. |  |

### Distension Cysts of the Follicular Apparatus

**Follicular Cysts.** May be single but are more often multiple; seldom grow larger than 3 cm in diameter. The cyst wall consists of an incomplete layer of granulosa cells, and outside that the theca layers of the follicle. Most follicular cysts are cysts of atresic follicles. Follicular cysts do not become malignant, and in most cases are of no clinical significance; but in cystic endometrial hyperplasia (p. 90) the ovary contains follicular cysts with an active layer of granulosa cells. Follicular cysts are common with fibromyomata, and in cases of salpingo-oöphoritis.

**Lutein Cysts.** (a) *Cystic corpus luteum.* The ripe corpus luteum occasionally becomes cystic, forming a cyst less than 5 cm in diameter which may be associated with temporary amenorrhoea.

(b) *Theca-lutein cyst.* Both the granulosa and theca interna cells lining a follicular cyst may become luteinized (without ovulation). The change is usually most marked in the theca cells, when the term theca-lutein cyst is used. In association with hydatidiform mole bilateral multilocular theca-lutein cysts occur, up to 10 cm in diameter, due to the excessive output of chorionic gonadotrophins. A similar change can be caused by clomiphene or gonadotrophins given to induce ovulation (p. 89).

Excision of follicular of lutein cysts is not recommended unless the abdomen is opened for some other reason. Haemorrhage may occur into these cysts, and they should not be mistaken for endometriomata. Occasionally intraperitoneal bleeding from a ruptured follicle or corpus luteum is sufficient to suggest an ectopic pregnancy and require laparotomy.

## Cystic and Solid Neoplasms: Pathology

**Mucinous Cystadenoma.** This is the commonest ovarian neoplasm. It occurs at any age, though most often between 30 and 60, and may grow to enormous size. The outer wall is dense and smoothly rounded, though rounded bosses may project from it. The cyst contains multiple loculi full of greenish-yellow slimy mucus. The loculi have a lining of very tall columnar cells, with uniform nuclei situated close to the basement membrane. Fibrous septa separate the loculi, and the epithelium tends to bud into the fibrous tissue and form fresh loculi.

If a mucinous cyst ruptures the condition of *myxoma peritonei* may follow, in which masses of mucin collect in the peritoneal cavity, and repeatedly reappear after removal. Such cases are probably due to dissemination of cells of the tumour.

The origin of these common cysts is still uncertain. A popular theory is that a mucinous cystadenoma is a teratoma in which one tissue outgrows other elements. Alternatively the tumour may arise from a Brenner tumour (see p. 74).

**Mucinous Adenocarcinoma.** On removal, about 10 per cent of mucinous cysts are found to be malignant. One part of a large tumour may appear malignant and another part benign.

In malignant cysts there is an area of solid white growth, usually adenocarcinoma. The growth infiltrates through the capsule to disseminate in the peritoneal cavity, and also spreads by lymphatics.

**Serous (Papilliferous) Cystadenoma).** Distinction is sometimes made between simple serous cysts and papilliferous cysts, but both have the same origin and nature. The *simple serous cyst* is thin-walled, unilocular, and seldom more than 15 cm in diameter. The cyst contains serous fluid and is lined by cubical epithelium. The *papilliferous cyst* is similar except that the lining bears papillary processes that project into the cavity. The papillae may be minute nodules or florid branching processes. Each papilla has a fibrous tissue core and a covering of cubical epithelium. In one-third of cases the cysts are bilateral; and similar cysts occur in the broad ligament (see p. 80).

If a benign serous cyst ruptures the fluid is quickly absorbed, but there is a risk of active epithelial fragments becoming implanted.

These tumours probably arise by metaplasia and invagination of the surface epithelium.

**Papilliferous Carcinoma.** About 15 per cent of papilliferous cysts are found to be malignant. In malignant cysts the epithelial layers are several cells deep, and the stroma is invaded. The growth penetrates the cell wall, and then becomes implanted in the peritoneal cavity, causing ascites, often bloodstained.

**Endometrioma ('Chocolate Cyst').** (See p. 81.)

**Dermoid Cyst (Cystic Teratoma).** These common cysts are sometimes seen in childhood, but most often during the reproductive period. They grow slowly, are usually less than 10 cm in diameter, and unilateral. At one side of the unilocular cavity is a projection, which is the essential tumour. This 'embryonic rudiment' is covered with skin, bearing hair and sebaceous glands. The greater part of the cyst wall is a fibrous capsule that encloses the yellow sebaceous secretion of these glands. The embryonic rudiment contains a great variety of tissues, chiefly ectodermal such as skin, hair and teeth, and less commonly other tissues such as bone, thyroid, gut, etc.

Dermoid cysts often have a long pedicle, and may lie in front of the uterus and are especially liable to torsion. Malignant change is rare, but squamous epithelioma may arise.

Teratomata are thought to arise when an unfertilized germ cell divides and proliferates for some unknown reason.

**Solid Teratoma.** These rare highly malignant tumours of young women rapidly grow to form a large mass with cystic spaces, consisting of a jumble of primitive tissues. One type of tissue may outgrow and obscure the others; for example rare tumours occur which appear to consist entirely of thyroid tissue (struma ovarii).

**Brenner Tumour.** This is a small solid benign tumour consisting of fibrous tissue in which isolated epithelial cell nests are scattered, and is thought to arise from epithelial rests which are normally found near the surface of the ovary. Some authorities hold that mucinous cystadenomata arise from the epithelial elements, and ovarian fibromata from the fibrous tissue elements.

**Fibroma.** A fibroma may be a small nodular growth involving part of the ovary, or the whole organ may be diffusely involved. The diffuse growths are often bilateral, and are smooth oval firm solid tumours with a homogeneous white cut surface. They consist of fusiform connective tissue cells, sometimes with some smooth muscle fibres. They arise from the stroma cells.

Though benign, fibromata are often associated with ascites, and even pleural effusion (Meigs' syndrome).

**Sarcoma.** This rare tumour is sometimes the result of malignant change in a fibroma or teratoma. It is a solid tumour, often with cystic degeneration.

**Granulosa Cell Tumour.** An uncommon tumour that arises most frequently after the menopause, but also both before and during the reproductive period. Its most striking quality is that it secretes oestrogens. After the menopause endometrial proliferation occurs with uterine bleeding. In children precocious uterine bleeding may occur. During the reproductive period there may be irregular bleeding or amenorrhoea.

The tumour is unilateral, solid and seldom large. It consists of granulosa cells resembling those that line the follicle. The cells are small, with deeply staining nuclei, arranged in columns or trabeculae, and often grouped in small rings. About half of the tumours are malignant, though not highly so.

**Thecoma.** A rarer type of oestrogenic tumour, consisting of cells resembling theca interna cells. Lutein change may occur in both granulosa cell tumours and thecomata.

**Arrhenoblastoma.** A very rare tumour that is found in young women, and secretes testosterone in sufficient quantity to produce virilizing effects including amenorrhoea, masculine growth of hair, breast regression and enlargement of the clitoris. It is a small solid tumour that may contain structures resembling imperfect testicular tubules. Usually benign.

**Disgerminoma (Seminoma).** A rare tumour, most often seen in young adults, also in children, occasionally in association with testicular feminization or gonadal dysgenesis (p. 26). It is a solid tumour of moderate size, consisting of groups of large deep-staining cells separated by fibrous septa. The growth is less malignant than seminoma of the testis, which it otherwise resembles. It does not usually secrete hormones.

**Carcinoma of the Ovary.** Carcinoma may start in the ovary (*intrinsic carcinomata*) or the ovary may be the seat of metastases from carcinoma starting in other organs (*extrinsic carcinomata*).

A. *Intrinsic carcinoma.* Usually both ovaries are involved when the case is first seen, and moderately enlarged into solid lobulated masses. Many microscopical varieties occur, but the commonest is a diffuse infiltration with columns of carcinoma cells (carcinoma 'simplex').

Three examples have already been described of malignant change in a pre-existing benign tumour (mucinous carcinoma, papilliferous carcinoma, and carcinoma arising in a teratoma).

Though some authorities claim that all such tumours are malignant from the beginning there is good evidence that benign cysts sometimes undergo malignant change.

B. *Extrinsic carcinoma.* May spread to the ovary:
(1) From other pelvic sources by lymphatic pathways or peritoneal implant, e.g., from uterine carcinoma.
(2) From distant sources, especially from carcinoma of stomach, colon or breast. The Krukenberg tumour is an example, and this arises from a small gastric carcinoma that may be symptomless. Bilateral solid nodular ovarian tumours occur consisting of a cellular stroma in which typical 'signet ring' carcinoma cells are scattered. It is possible that the malignant cells are directly implanted after floating free in the peritoneal cavity, but a lymphatic pathway is equally probable.

## Clinical Features of Ovarian Neoplasms

**Symptoms.** Uncomplicated ovarian cysts are often symptomless, and the first complaint may be of abdominal enlargement. Except in bilateral malignant disease some normal ovarian tissue remains, and menstrual disturbance is therefore unusual.*

Pain is infrequent with uncomplicated benign tumours, though large cysts cause abdominal discomfort. Pain occurs with endometriomata (see p. 81) and with many complications (described below): torsion, rupture, incarceration, infection, and with malignancy.

Frequency of micturition may occur with a pelvic cyst, or retention of urine if incarceration occurs. Large tumours cause oedema of the legs or vulva.

**Signs.** An intrapelvic cyst is found on vaginal examination as a rounded elastic mobile painless tumour, distinct from the uterus, and nearly always situated posteriorly.

Tumours large enough to be felt in the abdomen may be to one side at first, but come to occupy the midline as they

---

* Granulosa cell tumours and arrhenoblastomata are rare exceptions to this statement. Uterine bleeding may also occur with endometriosis (p. 81), or with torsion of a cyst, and postmenopausal bleeding may occur with malignant tumours.

enlarge. A cyst usually rises up out of the pelvis, but it may be possible to push it up far enough to palpate the lower pole abdominally. The tumours are usually smoothly rounded, though some are lobulated. The fluid consistency is obvious except in tense cysts, but in those a fluid thrill may be found. Ovarian tumours are mobile, unless large or complicated. On percussion the tumour is dull, and the flanks are resonant (except if there is also ascites) and no souffle is heard on auscultation. The lower pole of a large tumour can be felt vaginally.

The specific endocrine effects of granulosa and theca cell tumours and arrhenoblastomata have already been mentioned.

X-rays may show the outline of a tumour, and in the case of a dermoid cyst teeth may be seen.

**Malignant Tumours.** At operation, 20 per cent of ovarian tumours are found to be malignant, and clinical diagnosis of malignancy is not always possible. These symptoms are suggestive: Pain, rapid growth, postmenopausal bleeding. Malignant tumours are often hard and fixed. Ascites is usual, but also occurs with benign fibromata. Secondary deposits in the recto-vaginal pouch may be felt on rectal examination.

**Diagnosis.** Solid ovarian tumours may be confused with uterine fibromyomata, but the latter often cause menorrhagia, and are hard, multiple and attached to the uterus.

Ovarian cysts may be confused with the pregnant uterus, but in pregnancy amenorrhoea and breast changes occur, the pregnant uterus contracts intermittently, and cervical softening occurs. The retroverted gravid uterus may be confused with a cyst, but is continuous with the cervix, which is directed forwards. In difficult cases, especially when pregnancy and a cyst occur together, a hormone test may be useful.

With ascites there is a shifting dullness in the flanks, without a central tumour.

In fat women it may be difficult to exclude an ovarian cyst. With fat there is uniform resistance and dullness, and the umbilicus is deep.

The overfull bladder is certainly diagnosed by passing a catheter.

Inflammatory tubal swellings and pelvic abscess give

characteristic history and signs, and could only be confused with a twisted or infected cyst, though endometriomatous cysts can mimic inflammatory masses.

## Complications of Ovarian Neoplasms

**Torsion** occurs with moderate-sized tumours with long pedicles (e.g., dermoid cyst or fibroma) and is especially common during pregnancy or the puerperium. The cause is obscure. Torsion is often intermittent. The veins in the twisted pedicle are first obstructed, so that the tumour becomes plum coloured and swollen. If the torsion is unrelieved, the arteries then becomes obliterated, and necrosis and secondary infection of the cyst occurs. Tumours occasionally survive by acquiring a 'parasitic' blood supply through adhesions.

Torsion causes recurrent abdominal pain and vomiting. There may be initial shock, but later there is often slight fever, and sometimes uterine bleeding. The diagnosis depends on the discovery of the rounded tumour.

**Rupture** of a cyst may follow injury or occur spontaneously. The outcome depends on the nature of the cyst. Fluid from a benign cyst is quickly absorbed. Cells from a malignant cyst may be disseminated, or if the cyst is infected, peritonitis will occur. Rupture of a mucinous cyst causes pseudomyxoma peritonei (see p. 72). Dermoid cysts rarely rupture, but the contents are highly irritant.

There may be abdominal pain at the time of rupture, and subsequent events depend on the cyst contents. The cyst is not usually palpable after rupture, and with large cysts free fluid may be detected.

**Infection** of a cyst may occur by organisms from the bowel after torsion, from the genital tract after delivery, from an infected tube, or after the unwise operation of tapping a cyst. The cyst becomes an abscess, which may point into bowel or bladder, or may burst into the general peritoneal cavity.

**Incarceration.** A cyst may be held in the pelvis by adhesions, and cause urinary retention as it enlarges.

**Complications of Pregnancy.** Ovarian cysts are often

undiagnosed or misdiagnosed when associated with pregnancy. Complications are more common during pregnancy or the puerperium: torsion, rupture, incarceration or infection. The risk of abortion is slightly increased, and a cyst below the presenting part may cause obstructed labour.

## Treatment of Ovarian Neoplasms

Because of the risk of malignancy or of complications, all ovarian tumours larger than 5 cm in diameter are removed at once. Smaller swellings may be watched, but are removed if they grow.

At operation the whole ovary is often removed, but benign tumours can be resected, leaving part of the ovary. The risk of bilateral disease is high, and the opposite ovary is always examined, and in women over 45 should be removed if there is the least abnormality. Tapping of cysts is never justifiable, not even to shorten the abdominal incision, as the fear of disseminating malignant cells outweighs the slightly increased risk of hernia.

With malignant growths laparotomy is justifiable unless there is obvious remote metastasis. In operable cases ovaries, tubes and the uterus are removed. It has been suggested that the uterus may be left as a convenient cavity in which radium may be placed, but this is not the usual practice.

If there are widespread peritoneal deposits X-rays are unlikely to help, and cannot be recommended, but they are often used if there is a local pelvic mass which cannot be removed. Temporary retrogression may be obtained with various cytotoxic drugs, e.g., Chlorambucil 0.2 mg/kg daily. Dosage is controlled by observation of the blood count. Severe toxic symptoms and depression of bone marrow function may occur.

Tapping may relieve discomfort due to malignant ascites, but appears to hasten the end.

For torsion, rupture or infection, operation is required. During pregnancy ovarian tumours are removed, though it is justifiable to defer operation during the first 12 weeks for fear of miscarriage, and during the last four weeks if the tumour is above the presenting part of the fetus. Tumours causing obstructed labour are pushed up above the presenting part if possible, when labour can proceed and the cyst be removed afterwards; but Caesarean section is nearly always required, the cyst being removed after emptying the uterus. Tumours discovered during the puerperium are removed.

## TUMOURS OF THE BROAD LIGAMENT

### Wolffian Cysts

Kobelt's cysts, epoöphoric and paraöphoric cysts are described on p. 21. These are small cysts of little clinical significance.

### Fimbrial Cysts

These are benign, thin-walled, unilocular cysts that may become 20 cm in diameter. The cysts arise in the broad ligament between the ovary and the tube, and as they enlarge the ovary lies below them, and the greatly elongated tube arches over the cyst. The broad ligament is opened out, and the ureter may be displaced upwards. The cysts contain serous fluid, and are lined by cubical epithelium resembling that of serous ovarian cysts. They sometimes contain papillary processes resembling those in papilliferous ovarian cysts.

The name used here implies that the tumours arise from accessory ovarian tissue that is often found near the fimbria ovarica. Others hold that the cysts arise from junctional tubules or from the epoöphoron.

Large cysts are clinically indistinguishable from ovarian cysts, but when small are clearly unilateral and more fixed. The cysts are removed by enucleation, avoiding the ureter.

### Fibromyomata

Uterine fibromyomata grow between the layers of the broad ligament. Fibromyomata may also arise in the broad ligament or round ligament.

## Endometriosis

See below.

## Secondary Malignant Disease

Growths, especially of the cervix, may spread into the broad ligament and may obstruct the ureter.

# TUMOURS OF THE UTERINE (FALLOPIAN) TUBE

**Benign.** Papillomata and fibromyomata are very rare.

**Malignant.** Carcinoma is very rare. It is usually seen after the menopause and is often bilateral when first discovered. The tubes are distended with growth, either papillary or adenocarcinomatous. Early local and lymphatic spread occurs and the prognosis is very bad. The diagnosis is often missed, but bloodstained watery discharge occurs through the uterus, with pain, and the tubal masses are palpable. Treatment: when possible hysterectomy and bilateral salpingo-oöphorectomy, followed by deep X-ray therapy.

# ENDOMETRIOSIS

**Pathology.** The essential feature of endometriosis is the occurrence of endometrial tissue in ectopic situations. An 'endometrioma' may be regarded as a neoplasm, but will only survive under the influence of the ovarian hormones. The ectopic tissue consists of both glands and stroma, in both of which cyclical menstrual changes occur. The menstrual blood and secretion causes secondary proliferation, and the greater part of any tumour is adventitious tissue. Malignant change is very rare indeed. Endometriosis occurs in the following situations:
(1) Ovaries. Small dark endometrial 'spots' appear on the surface, and the menstrual secretion partly distends the endometrial glands and partly enters the peritoneal cavity,

where it is walled off by adhesions. A tumour mass is formed, consisting partly of ovary, partly of adventitious fibrous tissue, and with cystic spaces containing chocolate coloured altered blood. The disease is usually bilateral, and forms masses up to 10 cm in diameter.

(2) Uterus. Nodules ('adenomyomata') appear in the wall, resembling fibromyomata, except that they have no definite capsule and may show minute spaces containing blood. Microscopically endometrial tissue is found, with proliferation of adjacent muscle and fibrous tissue.

(3) Uterine tubes. Uncommon, except in amputation stumps.

(4) Recto-vaginal septum. A hard fixed mass of indefinite outline appears, and may extend backwards partially to surround the rectum. Ulceration of the posterior fornix may occur. The rectal mucosa remains intact for a long time, but ultimately rectal ulceration and bleeding occur. Lateral extension may involve the ureter.

(5) Round ligaments, both intra- and extraperitoneal portions.

(6) Umbilicus.

(7) Lower abdominal scars, especially after hysterotomy.

(8) Anywhere on the pelvic peritoneum. Fibrosis around endometriosis of the bowel may form a ring stricture and cause obstruction. The peritoneal surface of the bladder may be involved.

**Aetiological Theories.** Endometriosis only occurs in tissues adjacent to the Müllerian system. Various theories:

(1) Uterine endometriosis may arise by downgrowth from the endometrium. (Cullen.)

(2) Endometrial 'spills' may be regurgitated through the tubes and become implanted. The ovary may be a 'forcing-bed', in which endometriosis may grow, and from which further spills may occur. (Samson.)

(3) Endometriosis may be due to metaplasia of the coelomic epithelium from which the Müllerian system developed. (Iwanow-Meyer.) This may represent an abnormal response to oestrogens; fibromyomata, cystic endometrial hyperplasia, and ovarian follicular cysts are often associated with endometriosis.

(4) Lymphatic spread has been suggested, but the theory is not generally accepted.

**Symptoms.** Endometriosis occurs during the reproductive period, but rarely under 30. Small lesions may be found unexpectedly at operation, but larger lesions cause the following symptoms:

(1) Pain. Dysmenorrhoea occurs, and any palpable tumour may become more tender at the time of the period. Recto-vaginal lesions cause dyspareunia.
(2) Menorrhagia and irregular bleeding occur from associated endometrial hyperplasia or from uterine lesions.
(3) Infertility is due to pelvic adhesions or endometrial abnormalities. If pregnancy does occur, there is often considerable and lasting improvement.
(4) Symptoms of intestinal obstruction may occur.

**Signs.** Physical signs depend on the site of the disease:

(a) 'Chocolate cysts' are tender, fixed, bilateral masses; simulating chronic salpingo-oöphoritis, but without any history of infection, fever or discharge.
(b) Uterine lesions cause nodular or uniform uterine enlargement, and may be clinically indistinguishable from fibromyomata or from diffuse hyperplasia.
(c) Recto-vaginal lesions are tender, hard, fixed, and simulate rectal carcinoma. In contrast to carcinoma, rectal ulceration is rare and very late.
(d) Local lesions (e.g., in scars) may be tender at periods.
(e) Endometriosis of bowel may be indistinguishable from carcinoma without histological examination, except that there are often other endometriomatous lesions.

**Treatment.** In young women with severe symptoms, affected tissue is excised, conserving ovarian tissue whenever possible, although there is some risk of recurrence. In women over 40 more radical excision is advised, e.g. hysterectomy and removal of both ovaries. Recto-vaginal lesions may be difficult to excise, and the induction of the menopause by oöphorectomy or radiation may be safer. Presacral neurectomy is sometimes performed for the relief of pain.

Hormone treatment is probably only of temporary benefit. It was noted that improvement often occurred in cases that became pregnant and progesterones are given to induce pseudo-pregnancy. Dydrogesterone (p. 118) may be given in increasing doses up to 100 mg daily. This is continued for at least six months.

Chapter 7

# FUNCTIONAL DISORDERS OF MENSTRUATION

## AMENORRHOEA

Amenorrhoea (absence of menstrual periods) is *physiological* before puberty, during pregnancy and lactation, and after the menopause. *Pathological* amenorrhoea is termed primary when the patient has never menstruated; or secondary when the periods cease after having once appeared. Pathological amenorrhoea may be false (cryptomenorrhoea) when the flow does not escape because of some obstruction (p. 24); or true, when the endometrial cycle is absent.

**True Pathological Amenorrhoea** may be due to:

(1) UTERINE DISORDERS.
   (*a*) The uterus may be congenitally defective (p. 22).
   (*b*) The endometrium atrophies after irradiation with X-rays or radium, and hysterectomy obviously causes amenorrhoea.

(2) OVARIAN DISORDERS.
   (*a*) Failure of ovarian development occurs in cases of gonadal dysgenesis (p. 26).
   (*b*) Stein-Leventhal syndrome is a disorder of unknown cause. After some years of normal menstruation amenorrhoea occurs with hirsutes. Both ovaries are enlarged, contain multiple small follicular cysts with hyperplasia of the theca interna, and have thickened capsules. There is no evidence of any pituitary or suprarenal disease. The urinary excretion of FSH, oestrogens and 17-oxosteroids is normal. There is evidence to suggest that there is a block in the normal conversion of progesterone to oestrogen so that an intermediate androgenic substance androstenedione appears in excess. Surprisingly good results are obtained by wedge-resection of about two-thirds of each ovary.

(c) Arrhenoblastoma (p. 75) is a very rare cause of amenorrhoea.

(d) Irradiation or excision of the ovaries causes amenorrhoea.

(e) Ovarian infections or new growths *seldom* cause amenorrhoea as such processes rarely destroy all ovarian tissue. Amenorrhoea may occur with bilateral malignant disease or pelvic tuberculosis, but ill-health is the cause rather than ovarian destruction.

(3) PITUITARY DISORDERS. There is failure of production of gonadotrophic hormones in the following *very rare* conditions. The amenorrhoea is merely one aspect of a general disorder, and the gynaecologist is seldom responsible for treatment.

(a) Pituitary Infantilism (Levi-Loraine syndrome). The adult resembles a graceful child. No effective treatment is known.

(b) Pituitary Cachexia (Simmonds' disease). This is usually due to ischaemic necrosis of the pituitary gland, due to thrombosis of pituitary vessels after severe postpartum haemorrhage and collapse. Failure of lactation is followed by genital atrophy, loss of pubic hair, with weakness, anorexia, low metabolic rate, hypotension and hypoglycaemia. There is no pigmentation. Treatment with cortisone, thyroxine and norethandrolone (an anabolic steroid) may cause some improvement.

(c) Dystrophia-adiposo-genitalis (Fröhlich's syndrome) is characterized by dwarfing, adiposity and genital infantilism, and is usually caused by a craniopharyngioma that involves the pituitary gland and hypothalamus. Treatment is surgical.

(d) In acromegaly the eosinophilic adenoma of the pituitary gland may destroy the gonadotrophic cells, and the same may happen with other pituitary tumours.

(4) OTHER ENDOCRINE DISORDERS. Amenorrhoea occurs:

(a) In severe cases of hyperthyroidism, myxoedema and cretinism.

(b) In some cases of diabetes.

(c) In Addison's disease.

(d) With adrenocortical tumour or hyperplasia. Apart from cases of the adrenogenital syndrome (see p. 27) an excess of androgens may be produced in adult life by tumours or hyperplasia of the suprarenal cortex. With the amenorrhoea there is hirsutes and enlargement of the clitoris. There will be an excess of oxosteroids in the urine. Surgical treatment.

In Cushing's syndrome there is also cortical hyperplasia or tumour, but in this syndrome there is chiefly an excess of glucocorticoids. The patients are obese, often with cutaneous striae, hirsutes, hypertension, osteoporosis and diabetes. Surgical treatment may be possible.

(5) NERVOUS DISORDERS. Amenorrhoea is often due to emotional disturbance (e.g., fear or hope of pregnancy, or the stress of a new environment) and occurs in many psychoses. The mechanism is uncertain, but there are both nervous and vascular connections between the hypothalamus and the pituitary gland.

(6) DISORDERS OF GENERAL HEALTH AND NUTRITION. Any chronic or severe illness (including nutritional deficiency) will cause amenorrhoea.

(7) ORAL CONTRACEPTION. Temporary amenorrhoea may follow the use of the pill.

**Diagnosis.** During the reproductive period pregnancy is the commonest cause of amenorrhoea; otherwise *a local pelvic cause is rare.* In diagnosis general health is first considered, including psychological and environmental factors. Pelvic examination is essential to exclude pregnancy or uterine hypoplasia. Hormone estimations are theoretically desirable, and are now more easily obtainable. Withdrawal bleeding after administration of oestrogens proves that the endometrium is responsive. Ovarian function may be assessed by means of vaginal smears, a basal temperature record and endometrial biopsy. Pituitary function may be investigated by estimation of urinary FSH. If there is an excess of androgens the urinary oxosteroids will be increased.

In cases of primary amenorrhoea general examination,

This table summarizes the results of investigations in cases of amenorrhoea or failure of ovulation.

| | Menses | Endo-metrium | Urinary gonadotrophin | Urinary oestrogen | Urinary* pregnanediol | Urinary oxosteroids |
|---|---|---|---|---|---|---|
| Pituitary failure .. | Absent | Atrophic | Low | Low | Low | Low |
| Ovarian failure .. | Absent | Atrophic | High | Low | Low | Normal |
| Adrenal disorders | Absent | Normal | Normal | Normal | Low | High |
| Stein-Leventhal syndrome .. | Absent | Hyperplasia | Normal | Normal | Low | Normal |
| Cyclical anovular bleeding .. | Normal | Non-secretory | Normal | Normal | Low | Normal |
| Irregular anovular bleeding .. | Irregular heavy | Hyperplasia | Normal | High erratic | Low | Normal |

* There is a constant low output of progesterone from the suprarenal cortex.

careful assessment of the pelvic organs and chromosomal studies are required (see also p. 26).

**Treatment.** *Many cases of secondary amenorrhoea are temporary and recover spontaneously* but if amenorrhoea persists for longer than a year there is a risk of it becoming permanent. The principle of treatment is to treat the cause, whilst ensuring the best possible general health. Specific treatment is often disappointing, but has been outlined above. Thyroid is often given, but without exact indication. Cyclical courses of oestrogens, sometimes combined with progestogens as if to imitate normal cycles, often appear to restart the menstrual cycle in cases of secondary amenorrhoea. Also see induction of ovulation (below).

## HYPOMENORRHOEA

This term is used for a scanty flow, not for infrequent periods. The causes are those given for amenorrhoea, but a few women with normal fertility lose very little at periods.

## ANOVULAR MENSTRUATION

Sometimes in an apparently normal menstrual cycle ovulation does not occur and the endometrium does not reach the secretory phase. The frequency of the condition is unknown; it may be temporary or recur in many cycles. It is more common at puberty or near the menopause. Anovular menstruation is a cause of sterility; it is diagnosed from the basal temperature record and by endometrial biopsy.

*Induction of Ovulation.* It is possible to induce ovulation by injections of human pituitary extract (HPFSH) for seven days, followed by injections of human chorionic gonadotrophin (HCG) for five days, provided that there is a functioning ovary. There is no response in ovarian dysgenesis or after the menopause. The dosage must be exactly controlled by daily estimations of urinary excretion of oestrogens and preg- nanediol, otherwise dangerous bleeding may occur from haemorrhagic ovarian follicles, or multiple pregnancies may result. The supply of HPFSH is obviously limited. Extract of human postmenopausal urine (HMG) contains gonadotrophin and can be used instead.

Clomiphene is a synthetic drug whose action is not yet understood, but which will induce ovulation. Fifty milligrammes is given daily for five days, but again control by urinary hormone assays is essential.

## DYSFUNCTIONAL UTERINE BLEEDING

This term has been contrived to include cases of abnormal bleeding other than those due to complications of pregnancy or to 'structural' disease of the uterus or ovaries.

**Pathology.**

(1) In about a third of the cases there is *cystic endometrial hyperplasia (metropathia haemorrhagica)*. In this condition the ovary contains follicular cysts, but never recent corpora lutea. The follicles secrete oestrogens, but as ovulation does not occur no progesterone is produced. The continued unopposed action of oestrogens causes abnormal endometrial hyperplasia and hypertrophy of uterine muscle. The uterus is slightly enlarged, and the endometrium is thickened and elevated into polypoid masses. The epithelium is hypertropic, and many of the glands are cystic, so that there is a 'Swiss cheese' pattern. There are no secretory changes.

Either irregular or cyclical bleeding occurs, often after a preceding phase of six to eight weeks' amenorrhoea.

(2) In some cases the only endometrial abnormality is that secretory changes are slighter or less uniform in different parts of the endometrium than usual, possibly due to progesterone deficiency. Both excessive loss and shortened cycles occur.

(3) In a few cases bleeding occurs from an atrophic endometrium.

(4) In about half of the cases the endometrium appears normal, and we do not yet understand the cause of many cases of abnormal bleeding.

**Aetiology.** Often obscure; *many cases resolve spontaneously after a few cycles* and any claim that improvement is due to treatment must be considered critically. Presumably hypothalamic or pituitary function is at fault in most cases. Emotional disturbance can upset the rhythm. Pelvic congestion from infection or sexual stimulation may affect the ovary, and temporary menorrhagia may precede amenorrhoea in both hypo- and hyperthyroidism. It is convenient to discuss these cases according to the age of onset:

**Pubertal Cases.** The first menstrual cycles are often anovular, and ovulation does not occur, so that no progesterone is produced. The unopposed action of oestrogens causes endometrial hyperplasia and early periods may be profuse. Treatment: Excessive bleeding usually ceases spontaneously after a few cycles, and undue attention gives a child an undesirable impression of abnormality. Rest at period time and the treatment of anaemia are all that is needed. More severe cases may respond to 10 mg or norethisterone daily by mouth, during the last 10 days of the cycle.

**Cases During the Reproductive Period.** All the varieties of endometrial pathology described above occur, with either cyclical or irregular bleeding. Treatment: Sometimes patients give dramatic accounts of heavy loss which direct observation in hospital does not confirm; if the haemoglobin level can be maintained by administration of iron little else may be necessary. With severe bleeding diagnostic curetting is performed, chiefly to exclude other lesions, and it is also wise before complicated endocrine therapy. Curetting is primarily *diagnostic,* and if an endocrine imbalance persists the bleeding will recur. Any disorder of general health, anaemia, or any nutritional defect is treated. Rest in bed will often check excessive bleeding. Oxytocic drugs or ergometrine are of little use. Hormone treatment is frequently guesswork, and is often disappointing. Many methods are recommended; the following may be tried:

(1) *Continued or irregular bleeding without ovulation* may be treated with progestogens to induce secretory changes, and on stopping the hormone the endometrium is shed ('medical curettage'). Norethisterone 15 mg is given daily for seven days. Alternatively large doses of oestrogens (ethinyl oestradiol 0.3 mg two-hourly) may be given until bleeding stops. This is said to build up the endometrium

above the bleeding threshold. When the hormone is stopped withdrawal bleeding occurs, but often it is less severe. Subsequent cycles may be treated with progestogens in the second half of the cycle as in (2).

(2) *Cyclical excessive bleeding without ovulation* may be treated by giving progestogens in the second half of each cycle, e.g. norethisterone 10 mg daily from the 14th to the 25th day, with the purpose of inducing secretory changes.

(3) *Cyclical excessive bleeding with normal ovulation* is difficult to treat rationally or successfully. Some cases may be due to inadequate corpus luteum activity and these may be treated as in (2). In others, inhibition of ovulation may be attempted with oestrogens and progestogens in the *early* part of the cycle.

In exceptional cases surgical treatment is required. Hysterectomy is rarely necessary in women under 40, but is preferable to the induction of an artificial menopause in young women.

**Premenopausal Cases**. After ovulation and progesterone production cease at the menopause, oestrogens are still produced for a time, and their unopposed action causes endometrial hyperplasia, with excessive or continuous bleeding. This is a condition of limited duration, but its chief importance is in diagnosis; curetting is essential to exclude malignant disease. Some cases do not recur after curetting, but those that do are treated by hysterectomy, or occasionally by induction of an artificial menopause (p. 119).

## DYSMENORRHOEA

Dysmenorrhoea, or painful menstruation, is difficult to define precisely as many healthy women have some menstrual discomfort. Probably about five per cent of women have sufficient pain to seek treatment, and in about half of these the pain is enough to interrupt work. Dysmenorrhoea is of two types:

**Secondary Dysmenorrhoea**. Due to acquired lesions such as fibroids, endometriosis or salpingo-oöphoritis. Appears after some years of painless periods. It may be (*a*) congestive due to inflammatory disease or to endometriosis, or (*b*) less commonly spasmodic, due to uterine colic, while expelling fibroids or clot. Treatment is directed to the cause.

**Primary Dysmenorrhoea.** Far more common. It usually starts soon after puberty, though the first few cycles are often painless. The pain coincides with colicky uterine contractions (spasmodic dysmenorrhoea). It usually ceases after bearing a child, and is often relieved by dilatation of the cervix. Similar pain is produced by stimulation of the region of the internal os, when uterine contractions are induced.

*Aetiological Theories.*

(1) It is often stated that dysmenorrhoeic uteri are hypoplastic, e.g., sharply anteverted with a long conical cervix, or retroverted and retroflexed, and the proportion of muscle to fibrous tissue is stated to be lower than normal. There is little to support these views. Most dysmenorrhoeic uteri are normal in shape and size, and fertility is normal. Obstruction to the cervical canal is not now thought to be a cause of pain.

(2) Endocrine abnormalities: (*a*) The endometrium may be shed in abnormally large pieces, causing colic. Extreme instances of 'membranous dysmenorrhoea' occur in which the whole menstrual decidua is passed in one piece. Such abnormal shedding may be due to excessive progesterone effect. (*b*) When there is progesterone deficiency the uterus is said to contract unduly forcibly from unbalanced oestrogenic action. Against this view are the facts that pain does not occur in anovular menstruation or in cystic endometrial hyperplasia. It is now believed that progesterone stimulates rather than inhibits contractions of the human uterus.

(3) Prostaglandins from disintegrating endometrium may cause uterine spasm.

(4) Psychological factors undoubtedly accentuate symptoms, especially in a child who is led to expect menstrual disability; and in older girls there may be fear of sexual or reproductive abnormality.

(5) The actual pain is probably ischaemic, as the uterus contracts strongly enough to shut off its own circulation.

*Symptoms.* There is intermittent pain, which accompanies the flow, and rarely lasts more than a few hours. The pain is felt in the back and lower abdomen, sometimes radiating down the thighs. It may be severe enough to cause fainting and vomiting.

**Treatment:** The incidence of dysmenorrhoea in girls has been reduced by sensible education, by avoiding unnecessary restriction of activity during a period, and explanation of its normal significance.

Pain-relieving drugs are given in full doses, but habit-forming drugs are avoided. Phenacetin and codeine are popular. Pethidine is effective, but there is some risk of addiction. Antispasmodics are usually ineffective. Whatever drugs are used should be given in full doses. To restore confidence it is essential to break the sequence of painful periods.

The most effective treatment is to inhibit ovulation. This is possible with oestrogens alone or by using the contraceptive pill (p. 100), but the new synthetic progestogen dydrogesterone (Duphaston) is said to relieve pain without stopping ovulation; 10 mg daily is given orally from the 5th to the 25th day of the cycle.

Dilatation of the cervix under anaesthesia cures about one-third of the cases but this treatment carries the risk of damaging the cervix, and so causing miscarriage in a subsequent pregnancy. In exceptional and severe cases 'presacral' neurectomy is performed. Through a lower abdominal incision the hypogastric plexus is divided where it lies in the retroperitoneal tissue in front of the last lumbar vertebra.

**Intermenstrual Pain.** In rare cases abdominal pain occurs regularly at mid-cycle, presumably related to ovulation. Inhibition of ovulation could be tried. In very severe cases interruption of the ovarian sympathetic plexus by division of the infundibulo-pelvic ligament has been tried, but there is some risk of impairing the ovarian blood supply.

**Premenstrual Tension.** (See p. 16).

## Chapter 8

# DYSPAREUNIA, INFERTILITY AND CONTRACEPTION

## DYSPAREUNIA

Painful coitus. If pain persists after any initial hymeneal laceration has healed dyspareunia is termed *Primary*. It may be due to a resistant hymen, a narrow introitus, or very rarely to some congenital abnormality. More often difficulty is due to contraction of the perineal muscles ('vaginismus'), due to fear, resentment at previous painful coitus, or psychological aversion. With inadequate or unskilful sexual stimulation cervical and vestibular secretion is lacking, and soreness may ensue. Advice to the husband or the use of a lubricant may help. If there is organic narrowing or obstruction a plastic operation is needed (p. 121) or the patient may be given a set of graduated dilators to use. In the majority of cases emotional problems need discussion, and advice about contraceptive methods may be required. A psychiatrist can sometimes help.

If dyspareunia appears after previous painless intercourse it is termed *Secondary*. Treatment is directed to the cause, which is usually a local lesion, though it may have a psychological basis (e.g., a changed emotional relationship, or fear of further pregnancy). Pain at the introitus may be due to: Caruncle, acute vulvitis, Bartholinitis, tender perineal scar, kraurosis. Deep pain may be due to: Chronic cervicitis, salpingitis, retroversion in exceptional cases (p. 34), endometriosis, pelvic tumours.

## INFERTILITY

Because of the complexity of human reproductive physiology the causes of infertility are numerous.

### Male Factors

In about 15 per cent of sterile marriages the male is wholly at fault, and is partly at fault in a large number. The gynaecologist is not concerned with the treatment of the male, but only to know that spermatogenesis and coitus are normal. Seminal examination is essential. The specimen is obtained by masturbation or coitus interruptus, and kept in a glass vessel (not rubber) at less than body temperature during transit to the laboratory, which should be reached within the hour. A normal specimen measures 2 ml or more, and contains more than 60,000,000 sperms per ml of which more than 75 per cent are motile, and less than 25 per cent abnormally formed. Absent motility or numerous abnormal forms are more serious findings than a low count. Semen contains a ferment (hyaluronidase) that liquefies cervical mucus and the intercellular 'cement' between the granulosa cells around the ovum.

Alternatively a post-coital examination of the cervical mucus for the presence of sperms may be made. (See p. 97.)

Impotence, premature ejaculation and infrequent intercourse are obvious causes of infertility.

### Female Factors

**Ovulation**. Ovulation is clearly essential for fertility. Regular menses suggest regular ovulation, but anovular cycles can occur with apparently normal rhythm (see p. 89). Anovular cycles are frequent just after puberty, and become more frequent as the menopause approaches. In any severe illness or nutritional disturbance, or in specific endocrine disorders, ovulation may cease, and in many of these cases there is an abnormal menstrual cycle.

Local pelvic lesions will interfere with the escape of ova; for example pelvic inflammatory lesions, endometriosis, or (less commonly) other gross ovarian disease.

Ovulation occurs at about the 12th day of the normal cycle, though with variation from cycle to cycle, and conception is most likely with intercourse at or shortly before this time. Ovulation is presumed in a given cycle if an endometrial biopsy done just before a period is due shows secretory change. It is possible to obtain a fragment of endometrium without anaesthesia with a fine biopsy curette. In many women there is a transient fall in their resting temperature (recorded on waking in the morning) at the time of ovulation, followed by a persistent rise of $0.5°$ C.

**Transit of Spermatozoa and Ova.**

(1) *Vaginal and cervical function.* Spermatozoa soon die in the acid vaginal secretion, from which they escape by entering the cervical mucus. Incomplete coitus is therefore less likely to effect fertilization, and dyspareunia or vaginal obstruction may cause sterility. The female can conceive in the absence of orgasm, but sexual stimuli may increase fertility by increasing alkaline cervical secretion. Cervical mucus becomes less viscid at mid-cycle, when it is more easily entered by sperms; this change may be absent in endocrine disorders. In the pre-ovulatory phase cervical mucus crystallizes in a fern-like pattern if it is spread on a glass slide. Purulent discharge from cervicitis or erosion is inimical to spermatozoa, though conception often occurs in spite of discharge. After high cervical amputation, infertility may occur, not only because of increased risk of abortion, but because of altered cervical secretion.

The Sims test consists of an examination of cervical mucus within two hours after intercourse. If motile sperms are found then male function is clearly satisfactory, and any cervical factor in sterility is excluded.

(2) *Tubal function.* The ovum is normally fertilized in the uterine tube; obviously tubal blockage prevents conception. Blockage is usually due to salpingitis, including tuberculous salpingitis, which may be clinically latent. Salpingitis may not only block the tubes but also damage the ciliated epithelium. Pelvic adhesions from other causes may kink or bury the tubes, and they may be obstructed by uterine fibromyomata.

Tubal patency is tested by insufflation with carbon dioxide. (Carbon dioxide is used as it is quickly absorbed if it accidentally enters the blood stream.) Insufflation is possible without anaesthesia, but scrupulous asepsis is essential. A cannula is inserted into the cervix to convey the gas, which should pass through the tubes at a pressure of less than 100 mm of mercury. The passage of gas is shown by a rapid fall in pressure, and can be confirmed by abdominal auscultation.

An alternative and complementary investigation is by injection of 5-10 ml of radio-opaque medium through a cervical cannula, when the uterus and tubes (if patent) are filled and become visible with X-rays. The method is possible, though somewhat unkind, without anaesthesia. It has the advantage of showing the site of any block. Neither insufflation nor salpingography is safe if there is any active pelvic sepsis.

Laparoscopy (p. 129) is a most useful investigation, especially in cases of unexplained infertility.

**Embedding and Maintenance of the Embryo.** Ill-health, malnutrition and specific endocrine disorders will disturb the menstrual rhythm. Not only may ovulation cease, but the premenstrual preparation for the reception of the ovum may be inadequate. Commonly there is amenorrhoea or altered rhythm, but even with normal rhythm it is possible that in some cases insufficient progesterone is produced to maintain the early decidua.

Failure of embedding or early abortion may be due to local uterine disease, such as congenital hypoplasia, polypi, or fibromyomata.

In rats, vitamin E deficiency causes death and reabsorption of the embryo, because of interference with the yolk-sac placenta, but the human placenta is of different type and there is no evidence that human infertility is due to this deficiency.

**Investigation and Treatment.** In a young woman it is reasonable to wait two years before regarding her as possibly infertile, but in an older woman earlier investigation is justified.

General health and nutrition are first reviewed, and any fault corrected. A detailed gynaecological history is taken and the pelvic organs are examined. In a small proportion of cases gross abnormalities such as vaginal atresia, uterine hypoplasia, cervical fibroids, endometriosis or salpingitis are found and treated.

In the majority of cases no gross abnormality is evident and before proceeding further (or performing any operation solely for sterility) the husband is examined and when possible any fault is corrected. If he is at least partly fertile then the following investigations are required for the wife:

(1) Endometrial biopsy (just before a period).
(2) Tubal insufflation or salpingography (second or third week).

(3) Post-coital test and examination of cervical mucus (mid-cycle).

(4) Laparoscopy in some cases (p. 129).

If biopsy shows anovular cycles on more than one occasion, hormone therapy or treatment with clomiphene (see p. 89) may be possible.

If the tubes are occluded salpingostomy may be attempted, though the number of successes is small.

If cervical secretion seems deficient, oestrogens are tried, and an alkaline douche before intercourse may give the sperms a better chance of survival. Advice to the husband about coital technique is sometimes necessary, and about the timing of coitus in relation to ovulation. Artificial insemination of husband's semen is pointless unless normal intercourse is impossible. Injection of donor semen raises many legal difficulties, and adoption is usually a better plan.

Uncomplicated retroversion is probably unrelated to infertility, but sterility may occur in cases of retroversion with salpingitis or endometriosis.

## CONTRACEPTION

Advice on family planning is an important part of gynaecological practice. Such advice is not only for the benefit of the individual woman, but is of world-wide importance. If the present rate of reproduction continues the world population will double in less than a century. Infanticide is unacceptable; abortion is hardly different in principle, and is not without dangers to life and health; proper contraceptive advice is safer for the patient and cheaper for the nation.

Methods will be described in descending order of effectiveness. The failure rate is usually expressed as the number of pregnancies per 100 fertile women using the method for a year; e.g. for oral contraception 0.1, for the intrauterine device 2, for the diaphragm with a spermicide 6, for the condom and spermicide 8, and for spermicidal foam 24.

**Sterilization.** Although attempts have been made to devise methods of reversible sterilization these have had little success, and for practical purposes this method of contraception is permanent and is therefore only used for women with completed families or with medical contraindications to pregnancy. It is wise to obtain the written consent of both wife and husband before sterilization (or hysterectomy). The operation is performed by abdominal excision of the interstitial parts of the tubes; this is more certain than simple tubal ligation. Alternatively diathermy coagulation of the tubes can be performed at laparoscopy (p. 129). Rare failures occur from canalization of the uterine stump.

Vasectomy is often a good alternative.

**Oral Contraception.** This is a most effective method provided that the patient does not fail to take the tablets.

(*a*) Combined (Intermittent) Method. A pill containing a synthetic oestrogen and a synthetic progestogen is taken daily from the 5th to the 25th day of the cycle. The proportions of oestrogen and progestogen vary in proprietary preparations; the lowest effective dose of oestrogen is used to reduce the risk of thrombosis (see below). Minovlar contains ethinyl oestradiol 0.05 mg and norethisterone acetate 1 mg; Minilyn contains mestranol 0.05 mg and lynoestrenol 2.5 mg. (These are only mentioned as common examples; numerous other preparations are of equal merit.) If the patient forgets to take a pill she should take two on the next day. If a period does not begin within seven days of taking the last tablet the next course is started.

(*b*) *Sequential (Intermittent) Method.* A pill containing a synthetic oestrogen is taken daily from the 5th to the 19th day, followed by a daily tablet containing the same oestrogen and also a progestogen from the 20th to the 25th day. The method is claimed to have less side effects, but is less reliable.

(*c*) *Continuous Method.* A tablet of chlormadinone acetate (a synthetic progestogen) is taken daily without intermission, and without oestrogen. This is less effective than (*a*) or (*b*).

*Mode of Action.* Oral contraceptives inhibit ovulation and also make the cervical mucus more viscid. Cycles are more regular, and with less bleeding. Dysmenorrhoea may be relieved. Removal of the fear of pregnancy may increase libido, but fear or dislike of the pill has the opposite effect.

*Complications and Side-Effects.*

(1) Breakthrough bleeding. Persistent irregular bleeding requires investigation to exclude a pathological cause. If none is found it may be controlled by increasing the dose of progestogen.

(2) Thrombo-embolism. The risk of venous thrombosis is increased 10 times in women taking the pill over that in other women of comparable age, but the risk is still small. The mortality from pulmonary embolism or cerebral thrombosis has been estimated as two per 100,000, which is less than that from pregnancy.

(3) Liver function may be depressed, but this is unimportant except in women with hepatic disease or a history of hepatosis in pregnancy.

(4) Amenorrhoea may follow cessation of oral contraception, but usually recovers spontaneously after a few weeks.

(5) Cervical erosion is common. Moniliasis may occur.

(6) Hypertension.

(7) Migraine.

(8) Fluid retention.

(9) Nausea, but seldom for more than two cycles.

(10) Psychological effects are difficult to assess. Depression is often attributed to the pill, but seldom with much proof. Fear of the pill is common because of exaggerated newspaper reports of dangers. There is no evidence that it causes cancer.

**Intrauterine Devices.** These are made of radio-opaque plastic in various shapes that are intended to prevent their expulsion from the uterus. They are compressed or straightened for insertion through a cannula, without anaesthesia. A few women have menorrhagia and some have colicky uterine contractions. The device may be expelled, and some forms have a thread which projects through the cervix so that the presence of the device can be checked. It acts by preventing embedding of the ovum. A device may be pushed accidentally through the uterine wall during insertion; ill-effects seldom follow but it should be removed with the aid of a laparoscope. Infection and ectopic pregnancy are uncommon complications. The device has the advantage that the patient has no responsibility.

**Vaginal Diaphragm with Spermicide.** The 'Dutch cap' is a soft rubber diaphragm with a thicker rim. The rim fits the vaginal vault obliquely so that the diaphragm covers the cervix. The commonest size required is 70 mm diameter. Spermicidal cream, e.g. phenyl mercuric acetate (Volpar), is placed on both aspects of the diaphragm before insertion, and it is left in place for some hours after intercourse. The patient must be taught to insert the diaphragm correctly.

**Condom (Male Sheath).** A spermicidal lubricant increases security.

**Spermicidal Foam or Pessary.** An unreliable method.

**Safe Period.** At present this is the only method used by strict Roman Catholics. Since the length of cycles varies and the date of ovulation in any cycle is uncertain this is a most unreliable method, even if a basal temperature chart is kept.

**Coitus Interruptus** (withdrawal) is widely used, but is unreliable and may cause sexual dissatisfaction.

Chapter 9

# ABORTION AND ECTOPIC GESTATION

## ABORTION

Abortion is defined as the expulsion of the ovum before the 28th week of pregnancy. The great majority of cases occur during the first 12 weeks, when the whole ovum is separated by haemorrhage and expelled by painful uterine contractions. In later abortion the mechanism resembles that of labour; after rupture of the membranes the fetus is expelled, followed by the placenta.

### Causes

(1) *Fetal abnormalities:* The commonest cause of early abortion.
(2) *Uterine abnormalities:* Congenital malformations, fibromyomata, retroversion (only in cases of incarceration), deep cervical tears or amputation of cervix.
(3) *Maternal illness,* including acute fevers, chronic nephritis, diabetes. Syphilis causes late abortion sometimes.
(4) *Drugs:* Lead, ergot, quinine. (Purges and oxytocics, except prostaglandins, usually have little effect.)
(5) *Trauma.* Little effect on normal pregnancy, unless the uterine cavity is entered.
(6) *Hormone deficiency* (possibly).

### Types of Abortion

**Threatened Abortion.** Slight bleeding occurs, but soon ceases, and the pregnancy continues. The treatment is rest in bed, with sedatives if the patient is restless. Avoid purges. Progesterone is not advised except for some cases of repeated abortion (see below), as it is thought to stimulate rather than to inhibit contractions of the human uterus.

**Inevitable Abortion.** An abortion is judged to be inevitable when severe bleeding occurs, or slighter loss continues for more than about three weeks; when there is much pain; when the cervix dilates; or when part of the ovum is expelled.

In *complete abortion* the whole ovum is expelled and bleeding soon stops. In *incomplete abortion* bleeding continues and there is greater risk of infection. In a few cases the embryo dies, but is retained for some time—*missed abortion* (see below). Treatment of inevitable abortion: Give ergometrine (0.5 mg) intramuscularly. Examine carefully anything that is passed, to avoid doubt whether the abortion is complete or incomplete. Surgical evacuation is essential for severe or continued loss, and wise if the abortion is still incomplete after 24 hours. The cervix is gently dilated and contents evacuated with finger and ovum forceps or with a suction cannula under scrupulous asepsis. Blood transfusion may be necessary. Adequate rest is necessary after delivery.

Sepsis may follow any abortion, especially criminal abortion. There is pyrexia and foul discharge, and septicaemia, peritonitis, cellulitis or salpingitis may occur. Start chemotherapy with ampicillin while awaiting the bacteriological report on a high vaginal swab. If there is urgent bleeding, or if the uterus contains chorionic tissue, gentle exploration with the ovum forceps is wise, but all unnecessary manipulations are avoided.

**Missed Abortion (Carneous Mole).** Slow bleeding occurs into the choriodecidual space, raising hillocks of clot that project under the amnion. The embryo is killed but not expelled at once. There is a history of a few missed periods, but the uterus does not continue to enlarge. Slight bleeding may continue. Pregnancy tests may be weakly positive as long as any chorionic villi survive, although the embryo is dead. The risk of sepsis is small and spontaneous expulsion can be awaited. An intravenous infusion of ergometrine may be tried, and surgical evacuation is only considered after some weeks. There is a very remote risk of hypofibrinogenaemia.

**Repeated Abortion.** May be due to:

(a) Maternal chronic illness: including chronic nephritis, syphilis, diabetes.

(b) Uterine disease: congenital malformation, incompetent cervix.

(c) Fetal abnormalities.

Apart from these cases the term *habitual abortion* is applied to cases of repeated abortion with no evident cause. Hormone deficiency has been assumed to be a cause. Good results have been claimed after the intramuscular injection of 125 mg of hydroxyprogesterone caproate (Primolut Depot) twice weekly, so that slow absorption occurs. There is no very convincing evidence that this is effective, and with some of the other synthetic progestogens there is a slight risk of virilizing effects on a female fetus.

Since at least 10 per cent of pregnancies end in abortion for a variety of reasons, out of 1,000 women who each become pregnant twice, 10 women would be expected to have two successive miscarriages by mere chance, and would probably succeed in a third pregnancy even without treatment. Care must be exercised in studying habitual abortion series. Complete rest in bed (several weeks if necessary) is probably more valuable in preventing abortion than endocrine treatment.

Obstetrical injury or injudicious surgical dilatation may cause incompetence of the cervix. Abortion usually occurs in the middle trimester of pregnancy, with almost painless dilatation of the cervix and rupture of the bulging membranes. A torn cervix may be repaired before pregnancy; otherwise a purse-string suture of fascia or nylon may be buried in the cervic, either before or during pregnancy (Shirodkar's operation).

## INDUCTION OF ABORTION

Termination of pregnancy before the child is viable involves difficult ethical decisions. Some believe that the killing of a fetus does not differ in principle from the murder of a baby.

In Britain the Abortion Act (1967) permits termination of pregnancy if its continuance would involve risk (greater than that of termination):

(1) To the patient's life.
(2) To her physical or mental health.
(3) To the physical or mental health of the existing child(ren) "of her family".

(4) Pregnancy may also be terminated if there is "substantial risk" that the child will have such physical or mental abnormalities that it will be "seriously handicapped".

A certificate must be signed by two doctors, neither of whom need necessarily be the doctor who performs the operation. The operator must notify the Department of Health that he has terminated the pregnancy. The operation must be performed in an NHS hospital or a place approved by the Department. A doctor or nurse who has conscientious objections is not required to act.

Although it was stated in Parliament that abortion 'on demand' was not the intention, the Act is so vague that difficulties frequently arise. No method of termination is without some risk to life, health or fertility, and contraception is a much better method of avoiding unwanted pregnancy.

The genuine medical indications for induction of abortion are few and seldom absolute. The following are examples of sound maternal indications: nephritis which is progressing, malignant hypertension, diabetes with renal or retinal disease, carcinoma of the breast, and a few cases of mental disease.

Fetal indications are often less good, but termination has been performed for rubella in the first 12 weeks and some inherited diseases.

## Methods

(1) *Vaginal Evacuation.* The cervix is dilated with graduated dilators and the uterine contents removed with ovum forceps. This method is dangerous after the 12th week, but at any time it is easy to tear the cervix or perforate the uterus. A sharp curette should not be used. Haemorrhage is free, sepsis can occur and result in infertility from tubal occlusion, and evacuation is not always complete. Ergometrine 0.5 mg is injected intravenously at the end of the operation.

A better method is to aspirate the uterine contents with a suction curette after dilating the cervix. Before the eighth week a small plastic catheter can be used with minimal cervical dilatation and only local paracervical anaesthesia.

(2) *Oxytocic Drugs.* Syntocinon (or pituitary extract) is ineffective except in some cases of fetal death or hydatidiform mole. Prostaglandins are effective.

(3) *Intra-amniotic Saline.* Injection of 20 per cent salt solution into the amniotic cavity by the abdominal route usually kills the fetus and causes abortion. There is danger of sloughing if the hypertonic saline is injected into the tissues or peritoneum, and of electrolytic disturbance if it enters a vein. Urea solution may be a safer alternative.

(4) *Abdominal Hysterotomy* may be required of other methods fail. It has the risks of laparotomy and leaves a uterine scar.

Sterilization by tubal ligature or excision can be performed at the time of hysterotomy, but after vaginal termination sterilization is performed by diathermy of the tubes at laparoscopy.


## ECTOPIC PREGNANCY

The ovum is normally fertilized in the uterine tube. Embedding sometimes occurs in the tube instead of the uterus, and in extremely rare instances in the ovary.

### Aetiology

Mild pelvic infection (occasionally tuberculous) may damage the tube without causing complete obstruction, and so impede the onward passage of the ovum. Congenital diverticula may hold up the ovum. In many cases no cause is evident.

### Pathology

Tubal pregnancy is commonest in the ampulla, but may occur in the isthmus or interstitial tube. The ovum burrows through the tubal mucosa into the muscle wall, where its enlargement splits the wall into two laminae. The tube cannot hypertrophy to accommodate the growing ovum and eventually the gestation sac gives way with the following results:

**External Tubal Rupture.** The sac ruptures outwards.

(1) *Intraperitoneal rupture.* Usually rupture occurs into the

peritoneal cavity with free bleeding. Haemorrhage may be torrential, or slower when blood collects beside the tube (paratubal haematocele) or runs down to collect in the recto-vaginal pouch (pelvic haematocele).

(2) *Intraligamentary rupture.* Less commonly rupture occurs between the layers of the broad ligament (intraligamentary haematoma).

In both intraperitoneal and intraligamentary rupture the embryo usually dies, but rarely it retains sufficient chorionic attachment to survive as a secondary abdominal or intraligamentary pregnancy.

**Internal Tubal Rupture**. The sac may rupture into the tubal lumen. The ovum, together with blood clot, may be retained in the tube (tubal mole) or expelled through the abdominal ostium by muscular contractions (tubal abortion). In either case blood escapes from the ostium and may collect nearby (peritubal haematocele) or run down to the recto-vaginal pouch (pelvic haematocele).

In response to the pregnancy hormones, the empty uterus enlarges and decidual formation occurs. When the ovum dies the decidua breaks down and uterine bleeding occurs.

In the rare cases in which the fetus survives the placenta becomes attached to bowel or other adjacent structures, which become matted to the gestation sac. Fetal abnormalities are common. At term, 'false labour' (painful uterine contractions) is followed by fetal death. A retained dead fetus may become calcified (lithopaedion), or infection may occur with formation of an abscess containing fetal bones.

### Clinical Features

These depend chiefly upon the amount and rate of intraperitoneal bleeding. There is (1) usually amenorrhoea—one or two periods missed, seldom more, (2) always pain, and (3) after a few hours, uterine bleeding.

**Cases with Severe Intraperitoneal Flooding**. Although these cases are classical they are far less common than cases with slower bleeding (below). There is severe abdominal pain. The patient collapses and may faint or vomit. In severe cases air-hunger or even death occurs. On examination there is pallor, with a rapid pulse, low blood pressure and subnormal temperature. The abdomen is tender and distended (sometimes rigid). Since the tube has usually ruptured completely and the blood is still fluid, no swelling is felt on vaginal examination.

**Cases with Slower Bleeding.** The commonest type of case. One or two periods are missed, then persisting or recurrent attacks of pain occur with vaginal bleeding. Passage of a decidual cast is rare. The patient is pale and the pulse rate is slightly increased. The temperature is often slightly raised.

There is lower abdominal tenderness and guarding, and on pelvic examination a very tender swelling is felt in one postero-lateral fornix (tubal mole or a haematocele).

**Pelvic Haematocele.** A few cases are first seen with a large haematocele, although there is usually a history of several days' abdominal pain. Pallor and slight fever are usual. A large pelvic mass, of uneven consistency, is found displacing the uterus forwards and bowel loops upward. Retention of urine may occur. A pelvic abscess sometimes follows.

**Secondary Abdominal Pregnancy.** Very rare and often undiagnosed. There is a history of pain in early pregnancy. The fetus is felt unusually easily, and its position is often abnormal. The empty uterus may be made out apart from the gestation sac.

### Diagnosis

Cases with severe flooding are usually obvious. Cases with slower bleeding may be confused with:

(1) Uterine abortion. In these cases there is no tubal swelling; bleeding precedes pain and is more profuse.
(2) Torsion of an ovarian cyst. There is no evidence of pregnancy and the well-defined tumour can be felt.
(3) Appendicitis. 'Almentary' history; pyrexia; right-sided pain.
(4) Salpingitis. History of the cause; discharge; high fever; bilateral pain.

If there is doubt examination under anaesthesia is essential. If a mass is felt beside the uterus the abdomen should be opened. A needle may be inserted through the posterior fornix to test for free blood, but this test is unreliable. Laparoscopy (p. 129) is preferable.

## Treatment

In cases with rapid bleeding operation is urgent (salpingectomy). As bleeding often continues or recurs, much delay for resuscitation is unwise; transfuse and operate simultaneously. In cases with slower bleeding operation is less urgent. An untreated tubal mole or haematocele may absorb, but without operation diagnosis may be uncertain and there is a risk of further bleeding or infection.

If a pelvic haematocele becomes infected it may be drained vaginally, otherwise the abdominal route is better. For secondary abdominal pregnancy, laparotomy is performed to remove the fetus. If the placenta is much attached it may be left to absorb. Delay to allow the child to mature is hazardous, especially as the fetus may be malformed.

Chapter 10

# SOME GYNAECOLOGICAL SYMPTOMS

It is convenient to review some of these.

## ABNORMAL BLEEDING

Certain terms are used, often loosely: Menorrhagia signifies excessive cyclical menstrual bleeding. Hypermenorrhoea is sometimes used when there is excessive blood loss, and polymenorrhoea (epimenorrhoea) when there is shortening of the cycle. Metrorrhagia signifies irregular bleeding.

No classification of causes of abnormal bleeding is perfect; the student is advised to devise his own.

### Bleeding before the Reproductive Period.

(1) Rare neonatal bleeding due to maternal hormones.
(2) Precocious puberty, usually with no abnormality, rarely due to granulosa cell tumour.
(3) Vaginal trauma or foreign body.
(4) Rare cervical sarcoma.
(5) Rare bleeding in purpura or acute leukaemia.
(6) At puberty: dysfunctional bleeding (p. 91).

### Bleeding During the Reproductive Period.

(*a*) PREGNANCY (irregular bleeding). Always remember this as a possibility. Abortion and ectopic pregnancy.
(*b*) ABNORMAL ENDOMETRIAL BLEEDING (cyclical or irregular bleeding).
   (1) Inflammatory disease: Salpingo-oöphoritis. Tuberculosis.
   (2) Neoplasms: Fibromyomata. Endometrial polyp. Endometriosis. Uterine carcinoma, sarcoma, or chorionepithelioma. Ovarian oestrogenic tumours.
   (3) Subinvolution.

(4) Dysfunctional bleeding (see p. 90), including disorders of the pituitary-ovarian endocrine system and emotional disturbances.

(5) Rarely, such general disorders as mild hyperthyroidism and leukaemia.

(c) CERVICAL BLEEDING (irregular bleeding, often on coitus). Erosion. Polypi. Carcinoma.

(d) VAGINAL OR VULVAL BLEEDING (irregular bleeding). Injury. Retained foreign body. Urethral caruncle. Carcinoma.

### Postmenopausal Bleeding.

(a) FROM THE UTERINE BODY:

(1) Inflammatory disease: Senile endometritis. Rarely, tuberculosis.

(2) Neoplasms: Endometrial polyp. Fibroid polyp. Carcinoma. Sarcoma. Oestrogenic ovarian tumour.

(3) As a result of oestrogen therapy.

(4) Rarely in hypertension or leukaemia.

(b) FROM THE CERVIX: Erosion. Polypi. Carcinoma.

(c) FROM THE VAGINA OR VULVA: Retained foreign body. Senile vaginitis. Urethral caruncle. Carcinoma.

(d) FROM THE UTERINE TUBE: Rarely, carcinoma.

## VAGINAL DISCHARGE

The most practical classification is according to the nature of the discharge.

### Non-infective White Discharge (Leukorrhoea). *Causes:*

(1) *Pelvic congestion:* Pregnancy. Large pelvic tumours. Sexual stimuli.

(2) *Increased secretory surface:* Erosion. Cervical polyp. Submucous fibroid. Endometrial polyp.

(3) *Irritant douches or contraceptives.*

(4) *Disordered general health.* The precise reason for the discharge is often obscure; often there is lack rather than excess of oestrogens. In fact many cases vaguely attributed to 'general ill-health' will be found to have a local vaginal infection, e.g. with monilia.

*Treatment.* In pregnancy no treatment is advised, except zinc cream with phenol (1 per cent) if there is vulval irritation.

Any defect of general health is remedied; proper exercise is advised and constipation treated. Endocrine therapy is usually useless.

Remove any local cause if possible. Cauterize an erosion.

In other cases, douching (lactic acid 1 per cent) may be enough to keep the patient comfortable.

**Purulent or Muco-purulent Discharge.** Caused by: Acute cervicitis. Chronic cervicitis (with erosion or polypi). Trichomoniasis. Neglected pessary. Senile vaginitis or endometritis. In children bacterial vaginitis (e.g. streptococcal) is sometimes seen.

**White Semi-solid Discharge.** Caused by monilia.

**Watery Discharge.** Urine from a fistula. Liquor amnii. Carcinoma of the uterine body. Rarely carcinoma of the uterine tube.

**Blood-stained Discharge.** Causes: Erosion. Cervical polyp. Carcinoma. Senile endometritis or vaginitis. Incomplete abortion. Retained foreign body.


# URINARY SYMPTOMS OF GYNAECOLOGICAL ORIGIN

**Frequency.** Pyelonephritis, cystitis, calculus, tuberculosis, and benign and malignant tumours of the urinary tract require consideration in diagnosis, but causes more frequently encountered by the gynaecologist are:

(1) *Vulvo-urethral:* Acute vulvitis. Gonococcal urethritis. Traumatic urethritis ('honeymoon cystitis'). Urethral caruncle.
(2) *Cystitis.* Secondary to cervicitis or to prolapse. Following irradiation.
(3) *Pelvic peritonitis* with bladder irritation (salpingitis).
(4) *Pressure* on the bladder: Pregnancy. Pelvic tumours.
(5) *Carcinoma of the cervix* involving the bladder.
(6) *Post-operative frequency* due to cystitis, or to injury to the hypogastric nerve plexus.

**Incontinence.** *True incontinence.* Due to a ureteric or vesical fistula or rarely to neurological disorders.

*False incontinence* is retention with overflow.

*Stress incontinence.* (See p. 31).

**Retention.** *Mechanical.* Impacted pelvic tumours: retroverted gravid uterus, fibromyoma, ovarian tumour. Rarely due to pelvic abscess, pelvic haematocele or haematocolpos. Sometimes with procidentia. Urethral obstruction by stricture, calculus or new growth is rare in women.

*Nervous.* Post-operative and puerperal, from reflex inhibition and bladder bruising. Inhibition with a painful caruncle. Neurological disease, e.g., cord injury, disseminated sclerosis, tabes, hysteria.

## BACKACHE IN WOMEN

*A woman with backache usually has something wrong with her back.* In relatively few cases is a visceral cause found. A patient whose backache is caused by gynaecological disorder has additional gynaecological symptoms, or else definite pelvic physical signs. Pain referred from the pelvic organs is not felt higher up than the lower lumbar region. If movements of the back are limited or painful there is a local cause.

Gynaecological causes of backache include:

(1) Prolapse (occasionally).
(2) Retroversion seldom causes backache; it is possible in puerperal cases, or cases with prolapse or with infection.
(3) Inflammatory lesions such as cervicitis or salpingitis.
(4) Pressure from large tumours.
(5) Malignant metastases.

Postural defects and muscular weakness are common causes of backache in the puerperium. Rarely, sacro-iliac strain, symphysial separation or coccygeal fracture follow delivery, and a prolapsed intervertebral disc may date from that time.

The other multitudinous causes of backache will not be described, but may be broadly classified into:

(1) Referred pain from the renal tract, from other viscera, or from lesions of the spinal cord (rare).
(2) Pain due to local lesions of bones, joints, ligaments, muscles or fasciae (common).

Chapter 11

# GYNAECOLOGICAL TREATMENT

## ENDOCRINE TREATMENT

Many forms of endocrine treatment are still under trial and of uncertain value. Proprietary names for endocrine preparations are confusing and should be avoided whenever possible, but unfortunately the chemical names are often unwieldy.

### Gonadotrophic Hormones

These are glycoproteins which can be assayed in urine or serum by radio-immuno-assay in arbitrary units. The usual dosage is several thousand units by injection. Animal extracts (e.g. from pregnant mare's serum) have been used, but are ineffective as antibodies are soon formed against them.

Follicle stimulating hormone can be extracted from human pituitary glands obtained at autopsy (HPFSH). This has been used to induce ovulation (p. 89) but obviously the supply is limited. Extracts of human postmenopausal urine (HMG) also contain gonadotrophins.

Human chorionic gonadotrophin (HCG) can be extracted from pregnancy urine or placentae. Although it differs from pituitary LH it has some luteinizing action, and is used for this.

Clomiphene is a synthetic substance (related to chloro-trianisene) which has been used to induce ovulation.

### Chemistry of the Ovarian Steroids

It is not intended that the student should memorize the chemical details given in this section—their purpose is only to aid understanding.

Oestrogens, progesterone and androgens are all found in varying amounts in the adrenal cortex, testis, ovary and placenta. There may be a common biochemical pathway by which they are formed:

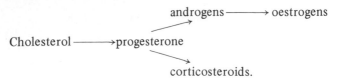

The cells of the adrenal, testis, ovary and placenta have specialized enzyme systems, and in each organ the common biochemical pathway is followed to a different extent. The normal adrenal chiefly produces corticosteroids, but oestrogens and androgens in smaller amounts. In pathological conditions (pp. 27, 85) an excess of androgens is formed.

The chemical structure of these steroids is shown below. Each carbon atom is given a conventional number, and some of these are indicated.

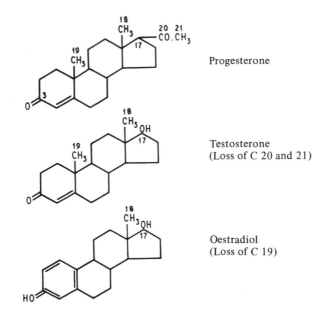

Progesterone

Testosterone
(Loss of C 20 and 21)

Oestradiol
(Loss of C 19)

## Oestrogens

The natural hormones (oestradiol, oestrone and oestriol) are relatively inactive when given by mouth and their activity is short after injection. Oestrogens can be bound to protein, so assay by competitive radio-immuno-assay is now possible. In urine, where large amounts are found, chemical assay is usual.

Synthetic modifications include *ethinyl oestradiol* with a $-C \equiv H$ group attached to C 17. This is highly active by mouth, as shown in the table below. Other synthetic oestrogens such as *stilboestrol* and *hexoestrol* are also active by mouth, but their chemical structure is unrelated to that of the natural hormones. Stilboestrol is cheap, but may cause nausea or vomiting.

After the menopause any oestrogen may cause uterine bleeding and serious diagnostic difficulties, and it should never be given without good reason. *Chlorotrianisene* (TACE) is a synthetic oestrogen which is given by mouth but is absorbed into body fat, from which it is released slowly. It is not true that it will not cause bleeding in postmenopausal women.

Oestrogens are absorbed through the vaginal epithelium, and are sometimes administered as vaginal pessaries.

Possible gynaecological uses of oestrogens can be classified thus:

(1) *Action on vulva and vagina:*
    (*a*) Vulvovaginitis of children (p. 45).
    (*b*) Kraurosis and senile vaginitis (p. 43).
    (*c*) Before colporrhaphy in the elderly.

(2) *Direct action on the uterus:*
    (*a*) Uterine hypoplasia is sometimes treated, but seldom responds.
    (*b*) 'First aid' for severe dysfunctional bleeding. Massive doses can be given to build up the endometrium above the bleeding threshold (p. 91).

(3) *Secondary amenorrhoea:* See p. 89. Oestrogens are useless for primary ovarian deficiency.

(4) *To inhibit ovulation:*
    (*a*) Primary dysmenorrhoea (p. 94).
    (*b*) Oestrogens are included in most contraceptive pills.

(5) *To inhibit the output of gonadotrophins* in cases of menopausal flushes.

*Approximate Dosage Equivalents*

|  | *By injection* | *By mouth* |
|---|---|---|
| Oestradiol benzoate .. .. .. | 1 mg | |
| Oestrone .. .. .. | 10 mg | 50 mg |
| Stilboestrol .. .. .. | | 1 mg |
| Hexoestrol .. .. .. | | 16 mg |
| Ethinyl oestradiol .. .. | | 0.05 mg |

## Progestogens

Progesterone is inactive when given orally but many synthetic progestogens have recently been introduced, most of which are active by mouth. Although all have some progestogenic qualities their actions differ from those of progesterone and may include some oestrogenic effects. A few examples are given below. Some chemistry is unavoidable.

(1) *Derivatives of progesterone. Dydrogesterone* (Duphaston) is a stereoisomer of progesterone. It has no oestrogenic activity, is claimed not to inhibit ovulation, and is of little use for treating endometrial bleeding. It is used for dysmenorrhoea (p. 94) or endometriosis (p. 84).

(2) *Derivatives of 17α hydroxyprogesterone.* If an OH radicle is attached to C 17 and a caproate group to that then we have *17α hydroxyprogesterone caproate* (Primolut depot) which is slowly absorbed after intramuscular injection. It is sometimes used for treating cases of recurrent abortion (p. 105). It has no oestrogenic activity, does not inhibit ovulation, and is of little use for cases of endometrial bleeding.

(3) *Derivatives of testosterone.* If an ethinyl group $-C \equiv H$ is added to C 17 in testosterone we have *17α ethinyl testosterone* (Ethisterone). This was the first progestogen which was active by mouth, but it is now used less as drugs of the next group are more potent.

(4) *Derivatives of 19 nortestosterone.* If the $CH_3$ group at 19 in testosterone is replaced by a H atom we have nortestosterone. If an ethinyl group $-C \equiv H$ is also added at C 17 then *17α ethinyl nortestosterone* (Norethisterone) is formed. Substances of this group have some oestrogenic effects, are potent in inhibiting ovulation, and are effective in control of endometrial bleeding. They do not produce an ordinary secretory change in the endo-

metrium, nor even an ordinary oestrogenic appearance, but an unusual type of proliferation.

Many of the contraceptive 'pills' contain substances of this group with a little oestrogen added.

The various progestogens have been used for treatment of dysfunctional bleeding (p. 90), secondary amenorrhoea (p. 89), habitual abortion (p 105), dysmenorrhoea (p. 94), premenstrual tension (p. 16), endometriosis (p. 84), and for contraception (p. 100).

**Androgens** have been used for the treatment of menopausal flushes (see p. 19).

**Thyroid** extract is often given but with little scientific reason to cases of amenorrhoea, dysfunctional bleeding, and of sterility.

## RADIUM AND X-RAYS IN GYNAECOLOGY

A. *In benign conditions.* An artificial menopause can be induced by X-ray irradiation of the ovaries, or by placing radium in the uterine cavity (100 mg for 24 hours, with screenage equivalent to 1 mm of lead). Besides acting on the ovary, radium produces endometrial necrosis, which may cause bleeding about a week after the treatment.

Indications: For some cases of (1) dysfunctional bleeding (p. 90). (2) Subinvolution (p. 49). (3) Fibromyomata (4) Endometriosis (p. 83).

The method is unsuitable for young women (in whom acute menopausal symptoms may be distressing), for cases with large tumours or much enlargement of the uterus, or in cases in which there is sepsis; and it should only be used when malignant disease has been excluded.

Smaller doses of X-rays have been used to stimulate the pituitary or ovaries, but the genetic hazard makes this unwise.

B. *In malignant disease.* Radium may be used for carcinoma of the cervix (p. 66), carcinoma of the uterine body (p. 69), vaginal or vulval carcinoma. X-rays or cobalt irradiation are sometimes used for malignant ovarian tumours that cannot be removed, in conjunction with surgical or radium treatment of other neoplasms, and for recurrences.

*Complications of irradiation.* (1) Anaemia and general toxaemia. (2) Burns of skin, bladder or rectum. Cystitis or bladder fistula, or proctitis with stenosis or a fistula may occur. (3) Vaginal stenosis. (4) Sepsis. (5) Acute menopausal symptoms.

## NOTE ON OPERATIVE TREATMENT

### Preparation for Gynaecological Operations

The date chosen for operation may depend on the menstrual cycle (e.g., endometrial biopsy). Repair operations are usually postponed if a period occurs, but obviously not hysterectomy for menorrhagia. The patient should be admitted at least two days before a major operation.

A general examination is made with special attention to oral sepsis, anaemia, the circulation and the lungs. The urine is tested for protein and sugar, and a catheter specimen is often required for microscopy and bacteriology. Cases of severe uterine bleeding often require blood transfusion. Operations that are not urgent are always postponed to treat any intercurrent ailment, including local sepsis, if possible.

The *rectum* must be emptied, if necessary by a saline enema before operation, but violent purgation does more harm than good, often increasing post-operative distention.

The *bladder* must be emptied before gynaecological operations. For major procedures the safest plan is to pass a catheter in the theatre immediately before the operation.

*Skin and Vagina.* Before abdominal section, the skin is purified in the usual way (Iodine 2.5 per cent, potassium iodide 2.5 per cent in spirit is recommended). Before vaginal operations douches are given if there is gross discharge, and oestrogens may be given before colporrhaphy in the elderly. The vulva is shaved, but 'painting out' the vagina is only effective with the patient anaesthetized.

*Anaesthetic.* No great subtlety is required. For minor operations pentothal is suitable (careful in the elderly). For major operations the usual relaxants are used. For pelvic floor operations many surgeons also infiltrate the tissues with a local anaesthetic solution with a little adrenaline. Extradural anaesthesia reduces bleeding.

## Vaginal Operations
### (Lithotomy position)

**Dilatation and Curettage.** Except in cases on intrauterine polypi and incomplete abortion, curetting is *diagnostic,* not therapeutic. Dysmenorrhoea may sometimes be relieved by dilatation of the cervix.

Procedure: After diagnostic bimanual examination a vaginal speculum is passed and the cervix is held with a volsellum. The uterine sound is passed, followed by a graduated series of dilators, until the cervix will admit the curette, which is used to scrape endometrium from the wall of the cavity. Forceps may be used to seize a polyp. Complications: Perforation of the uterus (see p. 30), sepsis.

**Operation to Enlarge Vaginal Orifice.** Procedure: Incision along posterior edge of orifice. A flap of vaginal skin is separated from the underlying perineal body. The perineal body is incised in the midline to enlarge orifice. The vaginal flap is sutured back to cover raw surface.

**Trachelorrhaphy.** (Cervical repair.) Rarely performed except for ectropion or repeated abortion. See Fig. 12.

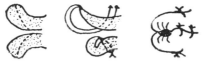

Fig. 12. Trachelorrhaphy.

**Amputation of Cervix.** Not often done, except as part of Manchester operation. After dilating the cervical canal the incision shown (Fig. 13) is made. The bladder is freed from the cervix and pushed up. The cervix is amputated and covered with vaginal flaps using catgut stitches. Complications:

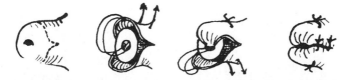

Fig. 13. Amputation of cervix.

Secondary haemorrhage (treatment hot douche, plugging, transfusion), stenosis, miscarriage.

**Excision of Vulva.** (Dorsal position.) The incision is shown in Fig. 14 and skin requires removal as indicated. Flaps undermined to allow block dissection of inguinal glands. Saphenous veins tied. Inguinal canal opened on each side and

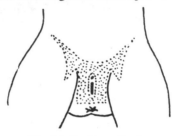

Fig. 14. Excision of vulva.

then the transversalis muscle is divided for extraperitoneal approach to the iliac vessels. The femoral gland of Cloquet is removed, and extraperitoneal dissection continues along iliac vessels to remove the iliac glands. Skin of groin sutured.

(Lithotomy position.) Vulva excised by incisions shown. It is possible to remove glands and vulva in one 'piece'. It is not possible to close raw area, which is left to granulate. Self-retaining catheter. Aftercare: Bathe down after defaecation, otherwise keep dry. Complications: Shock, sepsis, sloughing.

**Operations for Prolapse.** *Choice of operation:*

(1) For cystocele alone: Anterior colporrhaphy.
(2) For rectocele and deficient perineum alone: Posterior colpoperineorrhaphy.
(3) For uterine descent (usually there is also cystocele and rectocele).
    (*a*) Manchester (Fothergill) operation.
    (*b*) For selected cases of procidentia, or cases that require hysterectomy for some other reason: Vaginal hysterectomy with anterior and posterior colporrhaphy.
(4) Occasionally employed in postmenopausal patients: Le Fort's operation.

*Anterior colporrhaphy*. Essential steps: Draw down cervix. Diamond of vaginal skin removed to expose bladder (Fig. 15).

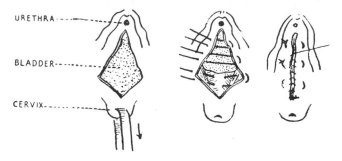

URETHRA

BLADDER

CERVIX

Fig. 15. Diagram to illustrate principle of anterior colporrhaphy.

Bladder freed from cervix and pushed up. Catgut sutures inserted to draw subvesical tissues together and close diamond.

*Posterior colpoperineorrhaphy* (Fig. 16). Essential steps: Dissect a flap of posterior vaginal wall to expose the perineal

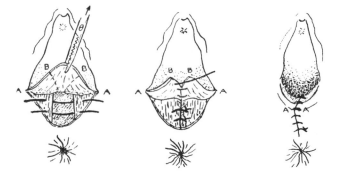

Fig. 16. Diagram to show stages of posterior colpoperineorrhaphy.

body. Suture the levator ani muscles together in the midline. Excise redundant vaginal wall, and suture vagina and skin. If the tear is complete, the torn ends of the external sphincter must be found and brought together.

*Manchester operation.* Essential steps: Incision as in Fig. 17. Excise diamond of vaginal wall, push up bladder and amputate cervix. The cardinal ligaments are now exposed and

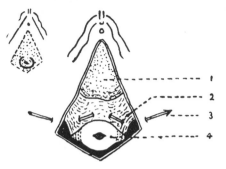

Fig. 17. Fothergill operation.

| 1. Bladder. | 3. Fothergill stitch. |
| 2. Cardinal ligament. | 4. Cervical stump. |

can be tightened by a stitch passed as shown and then tied. The cut edges of vaginal skin are drawn together to cover the cervical stump. Anterior and posterior colporrhaphy.

*Vaginal hysterectomy and repair.* Incision as for Manchester operation, but uterovesical and rectovaginal peritoneal pouches opened. The uterus is then removed after ligaturing the vessels in the broad ligamens on each side. The two broad ligaments, including the cardinal ligaments, are sewn together, and anterior and posterior colporrhaphy performed.

*Le Fort's operation.* A strip is excised from the anterior vaginal wall, and a similar strip from the posterior wall, and the two raw areas sewn together to form a vaginal septum.

*Aftercare of operations for prolapse.* Patients are usually allowed out of bed soon after operation. If a haemostatic pack has been inserted it is removed after 24 hours.

Retention of urine often occurs. A few surgeons insert a self-retaining catheter with closed drainage for 2 to 5 days, but most only catheterize if retention occurs. Sulphadiazine 1 g four-hourly may be given.

Avoid any local meddling; douche only if there is profuse discharge. Kep the perineum as dry as possible.

An aperient is given on the third day, and an enema subsequently if necessary. In cases of complete perineal tear the bowels are confined 4 to 5 days, and then opened with a small enema after instillation of olive oil or paraffin.

Catgut stitches do not require removal, but vaginal examination is made on the 10th day, when any abnormal adhesions are easily broken with the finger.

*Complications:* Shock (unusual). Secondary haemorrhage (treatment: hot douche, plugging, transfusion). Retention of urine. Cystitis. Minor sepsis is common but unimportant.

Care is taken not to narrow the vagina unduly if intercourse is still practised.

## Operations for Stress Incontinence (see p. 31)

## Abdominal Operations

**General Considerations.** The Trendelenburg (head down) position allows the intestines to fall away from the pelvis. Three incisions are in common use for pelvic operations. (1) Midline. (2) Paramedian. (3) Transverse suprapubic incision of skin and fat, which is undermined to allow longitudinal incision of the linea alba and peritoneum.

*Aftercare.* Nurse flat until shock is past. Deep breathing and leg exercises are enforced from the beginning. Morphia or pethidine usually required for pain. About 14 days in hospital, but patients are out of bed on the first or second day.

Encourage normal micturition, but if retention occurs and does not respond to carbachol (0.25 mg intramuscularly), catheterization is required, and sulphathiazole (1 g four-hourly) is given.

An aperient is given on the third or fourth day. If there is early distension, a simple enema is permissible, but irritant purges and enemas are evil. *Complications.* Treatment of most complications is the same as that employed in general surgery, and is not described here. (1) Shock. (2) Haemorrhage; primary, reactionary and secondary. Slow intraperitoneal bleeding may cause a pelvic haematoma; external bleeding may occur from the vaginal vault. (3) Sepsis; in wound, peritoneum or pelvic cellular tissue. (4) Urinary; retention, infection. (5)

Anaesthetic complications; vomiting, respiratory infection, lung collapse, spinal headache. (6) Acute gastric dilation, paralytic ileus. (7) Venous thrombosis and pulmonary embolism. (8) Late; incisional hernia, intestinal obstruction from adhesions.

Respiratory complications are less common than after upper abdominal operations, but femoral thrombosis and pulmonary embolism are common after pelvic operations. In most cases thrombosis starts in the veins of the calf and spreads upwards. Pressure on the operating table and subsequent lack of movement in bed are predisposing factors. In a few cases primary thrombosis of pelvic veins occurs, when operative trauma or pelvic sepsis are predisposing factors. Blood coagulability and the platelet count rise to a maximum 7 to 10 days after injury or haemorrhage; a common time for thrombosis to occur. Anaemia increases the risk. In cases with calf pain or swelling anticoagulants are used. Ten thousand units of intravenous heparin is given four-hourly for 48 hours. Dicoumarol or other anticoagulant is given (with the heparin) in doses of 300 mg on the first day, and 200 mg on the second. The further dosage of dicoumarol is adjusted to maintain the prothrombin level at 30 per cent of normal for about five days.

**Hysterectomy.** Apart from vaginal hysterectomy (not often used in Britain except in cases of prolapse) or Wertheim's hysterectomy (for cervical cancer), hysterectomy may be total or subtotal. In total hysterectomy the whole uterus is removed. In subtotal hysterectomy the cervix is left. Especially in parous women, total hysterectomy is best, as the cervix is often unhealthy at the time and may later be the site of carcinoma. Before the menopause, the ovaries, or part of an ovary, are conserved whenever possible.

*Total hysterectomy.* Catheter. Trendelenburg position. Midline or transverse incision. Broad ligaments (containing the ovarian vessels) are divided between clamps. If the ovary is to be removed, the infundibulo-pelvic ligament is divided, otherwise the broad ligament is divided medially to the ovary. The peritoneum of the utero-vesical pouch is incised transversely, and the bladder freed from the front of the cervix.

Uterine vessels are clamped and divided close to the cervix, avoiding the ureter. Vaginal vault is circum-incised, and the uterus removed. Clamps on vessels are replaced by ligatures. Vaginal vault is closed with sutures. The pelvic peritoneum is sutured and the abdominal wall repaired in layers.

*Subtotal hysterectomy* Similar procedure, except that the uterine vessels are clamped, and the uterus is divided, at the level of the internal os.

*Complications of hysterectomy.* As listed above, with the addition of fistula formation from injury to ureter or bladder. Secondary haemorrhage from the vaginal vault can be controlled by ligature of the vessel or plugging.

**Abdominal Myomectomy.** Transverse or midline incision. Some surgeons temporarily occlude the uterine vessels with a rubber-covered clamp that encircles the uterus at the level of the internal os, and also the ovarian vessels with a clamp on each infundibulo-pelvic ligament. The fibromyomata are 'shelled out' of the uterine wall. Incisions are planned to avoid the posterior uterine wall whenever possible, because of the danger of gut becoming adherent to posterior scars. Cavities left in the wall are obliterated with sutures.

*Complications:* As listed above. Convalescence is often stormy, as slight intraperitoneal bleeding occurs. Adhesions to uterine scars may follow. The operation may fail in that fibroids may recur or sterility follow.

(A polypoid submucous fibroid can be removed by *vaginal myomectomy*, by division of the pedicle after drawing the tumour down with a volsellum.)

**Operations for Retroversion.** Now seldom performed. *Ventrosuspension* (Gilliam's operation). Transverse incision. A suture is placed around the round ligament about 2 cm from the uterine cornu. A small incision is made in the anterior rectus sheath, through which a forceps is inserted, to pass anterior to the rectus muscle and enter the deep abdominal ring, after which it is directed along the course of the round ligament. By grasping the ligature the round ligament is drawn up and stitched to the anterior rectus sheath. The utero-sacral ligaments may be plicated at the same time. Pregnancy can safely follow this operation.

*Ventrofixation.* The anterior surface of the uterus is sewn to the anterior abdominal wall directly. This operation is never performed if further pregnancy is possible.

**Operation for Ovarian Cysts and Tumours.** Midline or paramedian incision. For large cysts it is better to make a long incision and remove the cyst entire rather than to withdraw it through a small incision after tapping, which may disseminate malignant cells. If the tumour is free the pedicle is easily clamped and divided. The pedicle is ligatured by a transfixion suture, and the pedicle is covered by drawing adjacent peritoneum over it. Adherent tumours are similarly removed after freeing adhesions, which may be a far more difficult procedure.

Benign cysts may be enucleated from the thinned-out ovary, or partial oöphorectomy may be possible. Even a small portion of ovary is worth conserving in a young woman, but in women over 45 the opposite ovary is also removed if there is the least abnormality.

If an ovarian tumour is considered malignant, both tubes and ovaries and the uterus are removed. The alternative plan of leaving the uterus as a convenient cavity for subsequent radium treatment is less satisfactory.

Aftercare and complications: As described above for any abdominal operation. There is a risk of an ovarian ligature slipping if the pedicle is not transfixed.

*Broad ligament cysts* are enucleated after incision of the peritoneum over them, taking care that the ureter is not pushed up and endangered.

**Salpingectomy and Salpingo-oöphorectomy.** If the tube is to be removed for ectopic gestation or to sterilize the patient clamps can be placed on the mesosalpinx and at the uterine cornu. After excising the tube the clamps are replaced by ligatures, which can be covered by drawing over adjacent peritoneum.

Operations for salpingo-oöphoritis are far more difficult. Adhesions are gradually divided until tube and ovary are free, when the ovarian vessels are controlled by clamping the infundibulo-pelvic ligament. The tube and ovary are removed, any other vessels tied, and raw surfaces covered with peritoneum whenever possible. If there is much 'oozing', drainage may prevent the formation of a haematoma which might become infected. Similar difficulties may occur in cases of endometriosis.

**Operations for Tubal Occlusion.** In cases of sterility, salpingostomy may reasonably be attempted if only the abdominal ostium is blocked. The tube is opened and the raw edges of the opening oversewn with fine sutures. Less than 10 per cent of cases are successful.

More difficult operations to excise strictures of the uterine end of the tube and to re-implant the tube into the uterus are even less successful. After such operations a fine polythene tube may be drawn through the tube, with the end brought out through the cervix or abdominal wall, and left in place for three weeks.

### Sterilization. (See p. 99.)

**Presacral Neurectomy.** Through a paramedian incision the posterior peritoneum just below the aortic bifurcation is incised longitudinally. The sympathetic nerve plexus is divided where it lies in the subperitoneal tissue in front of the last lumbar and first sacral vertebrae, taking care to avoid neighbouring blood vessels.

**Laparoscopy.** This is now a standard procedure. With general anaesthesia the patient is placed in the dorsal position with Trendelenburg tilt and her legs separated with stirrups. After emptying the bladder and placing a cannula in the cervical canal, a needle is inserted through the abdominal wall. The peritoneal cavity is inflated with carbon dioxide, so that the intestines are displaced from the pelvis. An abdominal cannula is then inserted to carry the light system and telescope through which the pelvic organs are examined. A separate small cannula can be inserted to carry a biopsy drill, or a diathermy electrode for sterilization by coagulating the tubes. Methylene blue solution can be injected through the cervical cannula; its escape will be seen if the tubes are patent. The patient can usually go home the next day.

# INDEX